NOTES ON MIASMS, HEREDITY AND NOSODES

Second Edition

Filip Degroote, MD

B. Jain Archibel s.p.r.l.
Rue Fontaine St. Pierre 1E, Zoning Industriel de la Fagne,
5330 Assesse, Belgium, Europe

NOTES ON MIAMS, HEREDITY AND NOSODES

First Edition: 1994
Second Edition: 2010
1st Impression: 2010

All rights reserved. No part of this book may be reproduced or utilized in any form or by any means, electronic or mechanical, including photocopying, recording or by any information storage and retrieval system, without permission of the author.

© with the author

Published by Kuldeep Jain for
B. JAIN ARCHIBEL S.P.R.L.
Rue Fontaine St. Pierre 1E, Zoning Industriel de la Fagne,
5330 Assesse, Belgium Europe
Tel.: +32 8266 55 00 • *Fax:* +32 83 65 62 82
Email: info@bjain.com • *Website:* **www.bjainbooks.com**

Printed in India by

B. JAIN PUBLISHERS (P) LTD.
An ISO 9001 : 2000 Certified Company
1921/10, Chuna Mandi, Paharganj, New Delhi 110 055 (INDIA)
Tel.: +91-11-4567 1000 • *Fax:* +91-11-4567 1010
Email: info@bjain.com • *Website:* **www.bjainbooks.com**

ISBN: 978-2-87491-007-4

DEDICATION

I dedicate this book to my ancestors, especially to the memory of my beloved father, Gaspar Degroote (1918 – 1972), who died at the age of 53 from cancer when I was 19 years old and I had just started studying medicine. It was the first indication because there is indeed a lot of cancer in my family on my paternal side.

The second indication was found in my personal history, because as a child I had a lot of typical features of the 'Carcinosinum drug picture' Foubister described, as whooping cough in three weeks old, in sleeping position, sensitive to music and fastidious. This made me clear that I belonged to the Cancer Diathesis and that I am the carrier of the genes that predispose to develop cancer.

The third indication happened to me when I was in Reichenau (Austria) to study the Mayr therapy. In June 1981, my 18 months old son had high fever. However, I gave him the most appropriate remedies with an interval of some days in succession, the fever did not subside and after five days I called Dr Pladys and explained him the case. I told him about the strong feature he had, that he only wanted to drink milk and refused every other drink or food. However, in the presence of that strong symptom, Dr Pladys, who was clairvoyant, advised me to give him Pulsatilla pratensis, which I did, and the next day my son was cured.

At the first moment I did not understand the prescription because Pulsatilla pratensis was not present in the rubric of 'Desire milk'. I could not ask Dr Pladys for explanation because he in the meantime was already severely ill and died one week later.

Then, some years later, I came in contact with anthroposophy where I found the description of distinction between ancestral and personal energy. The ancestral energy is the hereditary energy that comes from the ancestors and which dominates the personal development at the beginning of life. Whereas the personal energy is already present from the beginning and has to develop itself in such a way that it takes over the ancestral energy in the body.

So, it became clear to me that the symptom 'Desire milk' was ancestrally loaded, and its explanation was the presence of a classic nosode in that rubric. Then I separated the rubrics which contained the classic nosodes Carcinosinum, Medorrhinum, Syphilinum and Tuberculinum, and prescribed only, if possible, on the non-nosodal rubrics.

I started to study, more in depth, of Hahnemann, Allen and Roberts about miasms, and also the remedy 'Carcinosinum' of which I made a work which published in 1986.

Now, I stand 25 years later, where the incidence of cancer and degenerative diseases in my practice is nearly non-existing, thanks to the prescription of the right homeopathic remedies in succession, together with the intercurrent administration of the appropriate nosode. In that context it must be mentioned that Psorinum is the nosode which is mostly indicated as it holds the psoric miasm in balance and reduces, by the frequent intake, the connection with the individual remedy of the patient and the combustion of the basic life energy of the patient.

I am probably the only homeopath in the world who prescribes so often classic nosodes in connection with the individual remedy, I will explain how nosodes work on the vital energy and the miasms. I will also clarify how the use of nosodes makes the individual more free and how it stimulates the individuation process.

So, this is the story of the origin of fundamental ideas which contributed to the fundamental outline structure of this book and the way I practice. I wish you all an informative experience which I hope you can apply in your daily practice.

FOREWORD

A unitarian homeopathic physician should be considered good at his job if he succeeds to treat his patients for years, in 'all' circumstances and hereby keeping them in an optimal energetic balance of health by means of unitarian homeopathic remedies.

Generally it is rather easy to make a correct first prescription*. Real difficulties mostly occur later when the first remedy is not anymore effective and only few symptoms point to an exact following remedy.

In this way the less experienced homeopathic physician and his patients, who were both euphoric at first about the law of similia, will get deceived and may even forsake homeopathy. Only those who seek and study further will find the thread of Ariadne and unravel the clue, because in the end by treating problem-cases, one can obtain an insight into the dynamics of disease. In this connection the insights of Hahnemann and his followers concerning the chronic diseases are of vital importance.

The ideal way to heal a patient completely, would be the prescription of one single remedy, the simillimum, that would take away all the symptoms. Unfortunately, this happens rarely. According to literature this appears in less than 5 percent of the cases. The other cases require an administration of several,

---

*: The reason why a first prescription is rather easy to make is that this prescription can be based on the whole bio-psycho-pathology of the patient which is built up as a defense around the basic vulnerability, starting from the first impressions (mainly unconsciously) and first mental and emotional analysing.

This frame keeps upright till a first correct homeopathic prescription changes the inner tension and also its perception. So by its action the vulnerability of the person 'changes' so that the person can now change his defense and starts evolving which results in 'other' homeopathic remedies to prescribe.

more or less consecutive remedies. This knowledge is emanating from the first generations of homeopathic physicians, such as C. Von Boenninghausen, R. Miller, etc. Even Hahnemann advised to administer successively different homeopathic remedies in chronic cases (H § 171 and 215).

According to my experience **'psoric'** patients indeed react the to one fixed simillimum with an ease. But from the moment, the disease develops on a more complex miasm, a succession of several remedies is necessary to cure it.

I would outline, as clear as possible, the various pathways which should be followed. **Still, central to this method, a profound knowledge of the materia medica and correct selection of homeopathic symptoms, which lead to the correct remedy, is required.**

NB: The 'simillimum' is the remedy that, on the moment of the prescription, covers all the actual, valuable symptoms and consequently causes a positive energetic reaction.

F. Degroote, MD

PREFACE

When a homeopathic physician fails in the treatment of some of his patients, it is very instructive to get more insight the reason of this failure. Since years, I'm intrigued by this problem and I'm convinced that by obtaining a deeper insight, we can put a step forward in our therapeutic method. Hahnemann was also very concerned about this, and it finally moved him to formulate his ideas in connection with the chronic diseases. In my opinion there are two main reasons for the failure, apart from the low knowledge of the physician himself.

Firstly, there is an insight in disease from energetic-miasmatic point of view. By this means we have to recognize the hereditary and miasmatic load in our patient, from which we get a clear indication towards therapeutic approach. Moreover, the knowledge of the interactions between various homeopathic remedies is of vital importance. This book is dealing with that subject!

Secondly, the placing of our homeopathic treatment in a holistic approach is indispensable. Certain miasmatic (deep energetic disturbance) diseases can force the body in such an adapted condition, that this adaptation has to be corrected before the homeopathic remedy can unfold its action. This can be seen for instance where there are cranio-vertebral blockages.

Sometimes, a supplementary disturbing external factor can be present next to the actual miasmatic disease and attach itself as a layer upon the disease, so that first, it has to be distinguished and treated. This can be an electromagnetic disorder, an emotional fixation, an energetic disturbed area. Also, minimal nutritional imbalances can cause an energetic disturbance.

To perceive those problems, we can use 'kinesiology' which is a kind of body language, a method originating from chiropractors. To familiarize oneself with this method, it is necessary to study my book 'Physical Examination and Observations in Homoeopathy'. In this book you can find the description of the muscle tests cited with the chapters dealing with the nosodes, sarcodes and Bach flower remedies. By using this quoted control and affirmation technique, there is almost 100 percent certainty that our homeopathic remedy is correct.

PUBLISHER'S NOTE

'Miasm', the word itself has raised eyebrows of curiosity in the long history of Homeopathy. Dr Hahnemann introduced this concept with the 'Theory of Chronic Disease' after years of clinical research and experience.

Every new concept has its critical analysis by people who find it difficult to move out of orthodox thinking. Dr Filip Degroote's effort is again a step seperated from the league, as he brings clinically applicable concepts of miasm, heredity and nosodes.

Dr Filip Degroote has emphasized that in homeopathic practice the use of intercurrent anti-miasmatic remedy is very crucial. He has discussed all the three miasms and diathesis in detail. He has also discussed about the presentation, common disease conditions and different stages of the all the miasms. The psychological aspect of the miasms has also been considered. Cases have been presented which give a practical insight into the usage of anti-miasmatic remedies.

In addition Dr Filip Degroote has discussed about Bowel nosodes, importance of heredity and energy points. This work is a clinical necessity as it shall prove to be a beneficial tool on the desk of a physician for easy and apt references.

We trust this information will be found useful by all the readers and are sure if used appropriately, homeopaths will be able to achieve much better results in their practice.

B. Jain Archibel

INTRODUCTION

It is high time, in the world of classical homeopathy, that we can omit the 'trial and error' approach when prescribing a homeopathic remedy which we have been applying since the last two hundred years out of necessity.

We need a homeopathic prescription which is nearly 100 percent sure in regards to its correctness and efficacy. This certainty can only be obtained on the basis of a supplementary verifying method, which relies on a reproducible technique with a scientific basis.

Throughout the years that I have been in homeopathic practice, I have searched eagerly for such a technique and found it finally. I published those findings of that technique fifteen years ago in my first publication 'Physical Examination and Observations in Homoeopathy'. Because of the nearly 100 percent certainty concerning the correctness of the remedy to prescribe, this method has helped me over the course of years to collect more clinical material from my patients through daily practice.

There were three important steps in my development as a homeopathic practitioner, which can be compared with three successive insights:

First insight: In 1985, I set out and judged separately the nosodal symptoms, the hereditary energy rubrics in the repertory which contain Carcinosinum, Medorrhinum, Syphilinum and Tuberculinum and prescribed the individual remedy for the patient only on the non-nosodal symptoms.

Second insight: In 1989, I performed energetic examination by kinesiological principles. This results in the fact that the remedy which is to be prescribed can be verified to be correct even before being taken by the patient. Consequently, it accelerates the homeopath to get a deeper insight into the broad materia medica.

Third insight: In 1992, by administering the appropriate nosode[1] in connection with or shortly after the correct individual remedy, the case gains the momentum. The patient recovers more quickly from his acute or chronic problem, there is no homeopathic aggravation and there is a quick evolution towards a stable health.

The explanation therefore is that by administering the matching nosode, an energetic shield around the negative hereditary information in the chromosomes is formed, so that this information cannot be activated with the result that the energetic and physical expression of those bad genes will be kept dormant.

I am fully conscious that the content of this last proposition is actually so far rather revolutionary and will perhaps provoke a lot of reactions (or protest) in the present homeopathic world. Although already a large number of (especially Belgian) homeopaths have been trained in energetic examination and have come to the same conclusions. Only when the ordinary classical homeopaths make themselves familiar with the energetic examination, then they will also be able to come to the same conclusions.

---

1. A nosode is mostly administered on a complementary basis, when the simillimum is prescribed in a dose which has to be taken once only. Depending on the miasmatic background this can be, especially at the outset of the treatment, a classic nosode such as Carcinosinum, Medorrhinum, Syphilinum or Tuberculinum, or also a Bowel nosode. Sometimes this nosode is even followed by a (second) nosode, namely Psorinum.

    In the further course of the treatment it is a widespread classic experience that the nosode which follows the simillimum seems to be Psorinum. (cf. Hahnemann who compares psora with a thousand-headed monster).

    Thus, every time you prescribe a simillimum in the further course of the treatment, this will mostly be completed by the Psorinum. It is as if you can release every time the handbrake of the lethargic effect of the psora (as when you want to start your parked car and have to release your handbrake first).

    [**NB:** The administer of a trauma remedy, whether the trauma was physical or emotional, never requires to be succeeded by a nosode, because the disharmonious energy is not coming from within.]

This will consequently lead to the fact that, when we will accept this proposition as a hypothesis, we can practice in this manner 'classical homeopathy' at two different rates, namely:

1. **Most classical homeopaths** search for and prescribe only the individual (basic) remedy of the patient. Mostly this remedy originates from the mineral, vegetable or animal kingdom, and thus is not a miasmatic remedy which has a human origin.

> **NB**: The miasmatic remedies are remedies which have a human pathological origin and which are by their nature linked directly to the five known miasms. They include the following group of remedies: Psorinum, Medorrhinum, Syphilinum, Tuberculinum, Carcinosinum and Bowel nosodes.

By prescribing this homeopathically correct remedy, it touches (only) the personal energy of the patient, but not the hereditary energy. That's why the patient's complaints mostly improve, but the homeopath mostly misses the following **'awakened ancestral energetic disorder'** completely because this disorder cannot mostly be observed by symptoms. This gap now occurs for the present ordinary classical homeopath because they have no knowledge and experience with energetic examination. This 'awakened ancestral energetic disorder' is also mostly the reason why the patient goes through an aggravation. During this aggravation the patient produces known and/or new symptoms of the administered homeopathic remedy. The homeopath mostly adopts a wait-and-see attitude then. In that way the aggravation picture then disappears progressively as well as the original complaint. The disturbed buried ancestral energy which came temporarily to the surface has then finally returned again into a dormant state. In that way we, homeopaths, miss an opportunity offered to us to treat the deeper hereditary energetic disturbances.

We can see usually that the pattern of symptoms in this way of practicing homeopathy often keeps repeating itself in the future, as if the remedy was not able to effect a deep or complete cure. When the patient consults later again, they frequently find the previous remedy, which often also gain a repetition of the same reaction.

It is as if the patient wants to get out of a pit, yet can never really reach the edge and so falls down to the bottom again and again. That's why there's a high likelihood of repeating the (basic) prescription.

This results in a 'slow' energetic correction of the patient, by which the patient is not protected against his inherent tendency to suffer from degenerative diseases. This manner of practicing homeopathy refers also to the experience of Hahnemann who, after giving homeopathy for many years to his patients, had to conclude that his patients still suffered and died from the same degenerative diseases as people who had not been treated homeopathically.

2. **The energetically schooled classical homeopath**[2] on the contrary can diagnose this 'awakened ancestral energetic disorder' directly or fairly soon and can correct it by the most corresponding nosode. In this manner he avoids a (constant) aggravation with intensifying symptoms of the administered remedy, gets a quicker cure of the current problem of the patient and there is a faster cure of the case, and so there's a speedier evolution to a following complementary individual remedy.

---

2. How an energetically schooled homeopath works: First the homeopath has to be perfectly fluent in the method of the energetic examination (as described in 'Physical Examination and Observations in Homoeopathy') and has to be in a good balanced energetic state.

   Besides he or she has to consider possible disturbing influences of the direct environment (electromagnetic fields and rays) during the energetic examination. Furthermore, removable dentures and also the slightest metal on the body of both the patient and the physician must be removed (only during the energetic examination).

Introduction

It is as if the patient gets out of the pit in one movement and can evolve energetically right away.

This consequently results in a 'quick' energetic correction of the patient, in addition to which the patient is also protected against his inherent tendency for degenerative diseases.

How the common classical homeopath works

The Classical Homeopath interview with simultaneous observation of the body language, (external [physical] characteristics). After that he follows the evaluation of the obtained information which leads to a prescription. There is no 100 percent certainty that this prescription is the simillimum of the patient. This prescription is often 'trial and error'. In each case there is waiting for the reactions of the patient.

1. If the patient reacts insufficiently or not, the classical homeopath goes on to:
    i. Another potency of the same remedy.
    ii. Another remedy (!!! sometimes wrong).
2. If the patient reacts well:
    i. The prescribed remedy is the simillimum indeed.
    ii. The prescribed remedy is the only similae.

After administration of the simillimum, without administration in connection of the appropriate nosode, there is a fall back 'again and again' into the same energetic pit (which corresponds to a kind of an energetic standstill).

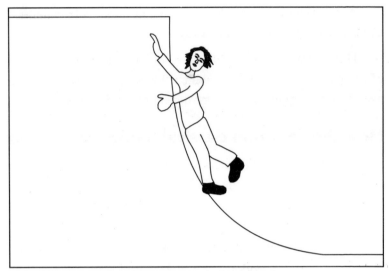
The common classical homeopath

How the energetically schooled classical homeopath works

The Classical Homeopath interview with simultaneous observation of the body language, external (physical) characteristics, etc. and then follows the evaluation of the obtained information and after that follows an **energetic examination** to identify the simillimum out of the selected remedy(ies) and to verify it. So, you are about 100 percent certain about the correctness of the homeopathic prescription.

It is striking that the energetically schooled homeopath also notices other energetic phenomena, such as:
1. Supervision in connection with the communication between both brain hemispheres.
2. Supervision over the dominating brain hemisphere: The energetic dominating brain hemisphere versus the congenital dominating brain hemisphere.

3. Which physical or energetic layer should be treated first (in order)
4. Which blockage can be present because of which even a good selected homeopathic remedy does not work. Such blockages can be:
   - Switching (breakdown in communications between both brain hemispheres), by which the prescribed simillimum sometimes cannot start to work
   - A classic nosode (Psorinum, Medorrhinum, Carcinosinum, Tuberculinum, Syphilinum and all Bowel nosodes), which balances the ancestral energy and makes the prescribed remedy work more deeply
   - Trauma (emotional or physical trauma, vaccination, etc)
   - Isopathic nosodes (nosodal therapy with virus, bacteria, fungi)

When these blockages are directly recognized and corrected, the right prescription can also directly affect deeply.

Many energetically working homeopaths ascertain that the interaction of the individual remedy (simillimum) of the patient 'directly' brings an ancestral energetic layer to the surface.

An almost simultaneous treatment of these ancestral layer (classic nosode), directly after correction of the individual energetic disturbance by administering the simillimum, will therefore bring an accelerated action and a greater profundity of the action of this simillimum.

In practice this can be done in two ways:
1. The simillimum is taken together with the nosode: While administering both remedies at the same time, the patient (with eyes open) is not allowed to blink because this opens an energetic valve between the individual energetic channels (the

10 acupuncture meridians) and the ancestral energetic channels (for instance the miscellaneous meridians, the governing vessel and the conception vessel). When these valves open by blinking while administering, then the energetic signal does not reach its destination. It has to be administered again and repaired after an interval of half an hour.

2. Or, let the patient take his simillimum first, followed by, at least half an hour later, the ancestral remedy (nosode) and this is the most easy way of administering.

By correction of above mentioned blockages and correction of the ancestral energy, we also see that the patient reacts quickly and also that the homeopathic remedy can bring change quickly.

When the simillimum is followed by the administration of the appropriate nosode there will be no fall back again and again into the same energetic pit but on the contrary the patient comes completely out and gets the possibility to further energetic evolution.

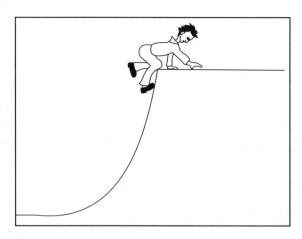

The energetically schooled classical homeopath

PROLOGUE

First edition

Although the use of nosodes in homeopathic treatment is generally approved, there have been no clear rules for their application so far.

In this book, Filip Degroote, known for more than ten years on account of his knowledge of the nosodes, explains the insight of nosodal therapy, heredity and miasms in a way it had never been told before. Concerning on classic nosodes, he differentiates the patient's symptoms into two groups: symptoms of the classic nosode and the individual symptoms of the patient. He advises to put aside the nosodal symptoms in order to recognize a more definite picture of the patient. The prescription of the nosode might be necessary in the future, or in an acute state, or when there is no progress in a case anymore.

Furthermore, for each remedy he describes the confirmatory muscle-tests, a working method he had already introduced in his book 'Physical Examination and Observations in Homoeopathy'.

Jan Sijmons, MD

Second edition

This second edition is totally a revised and enlarged edition wherein the author has put the accent on the development and understanding of the homeopathic chronic miasms.

He starts the book by the history of miasm from the time before Hahnemann till now. So, we see the change of the meaning of miasm from material into energetic, linked to the vital force.

So, Hahnemann was the first to consider miasms as the fundamental energetic cause of chronic diseases, which created a split with the ideas of the conventional medicine. Later on, new layers were added in the miasm theory by some eminent homeopaths, namely Allen, Paschero, Masi and others.

In this book, the author investigates on the psychological aspect of each miasm and diathesis. He explains the psora as a 'dynamic exchange' inside the patient between the self with its collective unconscious and the super ego. He deals with the many generations of homeopaths who tend to prescribe different homoeopathic remedies in succession. So, for him psora is not a static state corresponding to only one single remedy which will be suitable lifelong for that patient.

Furthermore, he has proved by his 25 years experience that besides the simillimum often the supplementary administration of the indicated classic, bowel or some isopathic nosode can cure right from the core and in the most effective way the involved miasm which he considers is the carrier of some negative ancestral energy. These insights are illustrated through the book by many cases.

Suzanne Van Rampelbergh, MD

ABBREVIATIONS

H	:	Hahnemann, S.: Organon of Medicine
H-CD	:	Hahnemann, S.: The Chronic Diseases
A-I	:	Allen, J. Henry: The Chronic Miasms, Vol. I: Psora and Pseudo-psora
A-II	:	Allen, J. Henry: The Chronic Miasms, Vol. II: Sycosis
m.	:	Muscle
Number	:	Radionic rate / code number corresponding to the preceding remedy
MD	:	Handmode (of the energetic examination)

- NB : Figure with the specific finger positions concerning the handmodes, see last page
- \- : Flexed (finger)
- O : Open (finger)
- T : Thumb
- I : Index / Forefinger
- M : Middle finger
- R : Ring finger
- L : Little finger

TL	:	Therapy Localization
Asterisk (*)	:	Additions by the author

CONTENTS

Dedication   *iii*
Foreword   *v*
Preface   *vii*
Publisher's Note   *ix*
Introduction   *xi*
Prologue   *xix*
Abbreviations   *xxi*

Chapters

1. **Miasms** 1
   - Introduction   1
   - Classic Miasms   5
   - Bowel Nosodes and Miasms   25
   - Work Procedure Skeleton   30
   - Cases (Illustrations)   32
   - Conclusion   38

2. **Miasms and their Psychological Background** 41
   - Miasms seen from Psychological Perspective   41

3. **Heredity** 53
   - Ancestral Energy   53
   - Diagnosis   57
   - Treatment   61

4. **Heredity and Classic Nosodes** 71
   - What Happens from Conception until the Development to a Grown Human Being   74
   - Conclusion   77
   - Cases   80

5. **Nosodes** 89
   - Definition   89

- History 89
- Indications to Prescribe a Nosode 90

6. **Classic Nosodes** 91
   - Screening of the Classic Nosodes by Energetic Points 96
   - Peculiar Features of Classic Nosodes 100
   - Common Features of Ancestral Energy out of Balance 114

7. **Bowel Nosodes** 131
   - Judgement of the Action of a Bowel Nosode 134
   - Bowel nosodes and their Related Remedies 136

8. **Psora and Nosodes** 163
   - Energetic Screening of the Psoric Nosodes by their Energetic Points 165
   - Work Skeleton to Identify the Specific Nosode ... 167

9. **What Happens when the Interaction between the Individual Remedy and the Nosode Starts** 171

10. **Isopathic Nosodes** 175
    - Monera and Yeasts 175
    - Energetic Examination, Muscle Tests and Energetic Features of Isopathic Nosodes 179
    - Relationship between Muscle Tests and some Homoepathic Remedies of Bacterial, Viral and Mycotic Origin 207
    - Conclusion 215

Appendix
   - Handmode Figures 217

Bibliography 219

Index of Cases 223

Chapter 1

Miasms

INTRODUCTION

Origin of the words 'Miasm' and 'Diathesis'

Miasm stems from the Greek word for *'pollution'*, *'stain'*, *'to pollute'*.

Diathesis stems from the Greek word for *'arrangement'*, *'disposition'*.

Miasma

Noxious exhalations from putrescent organic matter, poisonous effluvia or germs polluting the atmosphere.

A dangerous, foreboding or death like influence or atmosphere including a thick vaporous atmosphere or emanation.

A poisonous atmosphere formerly thought to rise from swamps and putrid matter and to cause diseases.

A poisonous vapour or mist believed to be made up of particles from decomposing material (from dead bodies or excrements) that could cause disease and could be identified by its foul smell.

Diathesis

A constitution or condition of the body which makes the tissues react in special ways to certain extrinsic stimuli and thus tends to make the person more susceptible to certain diseases (Dictionary of Cell and Molecular Biology).

Diathesis is an elegant term for a predisposition or tendency. For example, a haemorrhagic diathesis is nothing more than a bleeding tendency (Medical Dictionary – Webster's New World).

Miasma and miasm theory of disease

The Miasma theory is an explanation of the origin of epidemics, based on the notion that they were caused by bad smelling air, for example, emanating from rotten vegetation in marshes or swamps. (Websters Dictionary, 1998)

The Miasm theory of disease or Bad Air theory began in the middle age and continued upto the mid of the 19th century, when it was used to explain the spread of cholera in London and Paris.

In 1350, plague infested Europe as well as the Middle East, North Africa and Asia, making an innumerable amount of victims, the miasma was considered as the cause of that disease and this miasma was again the consequence of the positioning of the planets. Physicians at the Sorbonne university of Paris calculated that the plague of that time was due to the standing in line of the planets Saturn, Jupiter and Mars. By their positioning, the air on earth was becoming warmer which gave origin to the miasma causing the plague.

During the great plague of 1665, physicians wore masks filled with sweet smelling flowers to keep the poisonous miasma out. Because of the miasma, they sanitized some buildings, removed night soil from public proximity and had swamps drained to get rid of the bad smell.

Dr William Farr, the assistant commissioner of the 1851 London Census was an important supporter of the miasma theory. He believed that cholera was transmitted by air and that there was a deadly concentration of miasma near the bank of River Thames. The disease was said to be preventable by cleansing and scouring of the body and items.

Another proponent of the Miasma theory was the Crimean War nurse, Florence Nightingale (1820-1910), who was famous for her work in making hospitals clean, fresh and airy.

She wrote that 'the very first canon of nursing . . . the first essential to the patient, without which all the rest you can do for him is as nothing . . . is to keep the air he breathes as pure as the external air.' Foul air was the most important cause of infection.

From miasma to germ

Although the Miasma theory, because of its emphasis on odour, proved incorrect, it represented some recognition of the relation between filth and disease. So, it encouraged cleanliness and paved the way for public health reform.

The Miasma theory also helped to interest scientists in decaying matter and led eventually to the identification of microbes as agents of infectious disease instead of stench alone.

The clash of the old-fashioned Miasma theories and the developing new science did not lead to the defeat of the former and victory for the latter, but it conjoined the filth and the germs.

Miasm from homeopathic view

Hahnemann defines the 'miasm' as the fundamental energetic

cause of disease. Yet he created confusion by using the word miasm for 'nosologic entities'.

When Hahnemann found a disease, having always the same cause or always the same lesion or always the same symptoms, he named the nosologic entity as 'miasm'.

Then, at a certain moment he found 'psora', of which he said it is a morbid disorder of the vital force, which he also called 'miasm'. So, energetic as well as nosologic entities are called miasm.

> **NB:** 'I prefer to use the word miasm for the acute miasm and the three classic miasms of Hahnemann: Psora, Sycosis and Syphilis; when I discuss mixed miasms, the term 'diathesis' will normally be used.'

CLASSIC MIASMS

Nowadays, there is hardly any homeopathic school which applies the doctrine of the miasm as S. Hahnemann and H.C. Allen did. By the application of some modern psycho-analytic methods, a whole new movement has been created which ignore the insight of our founders. Nevertheless, every disease has a miasmatic background, and it is worth to consider it.

Hahnemann defines 'miasm' as an energetic disorder of the vital force which gives rise to the fundamental, constitutional and pathological state of the individual.

The entire psychophysical constitution of the patient is altered by this dynamic morbid tendency. Each individual is predisposed to certain specific diseases and to various perturbations with their own character and modalities.

Miasm is a term comparable to diathesis, dyscrasia, constitution or terrain. Hahnemann recognized three miasms, which he called Psora, Sycosis and Syphilis (aside from the acute miasm).

What is a disease?

The essential factor in the disease is an ethereal force or vibratory state, whether it is extrinsic or intrinsic. An infection, as a factor of disease, is essentially an ethereal force which can act directly upon a susceptible living cell, because infection is possible without the agency of any material substance or living cell. It is also true that infection is often carried by an infective organism, which is a postulate of Koch. So, the theories of Hahnemann and Koch are not really in opposition. But the most important factor in disease is the inherent susceptibility of each body cell, which is partly of hereditary origin.

In **Psora**, the typical symptom complex has reference to the skin, the basic epidermal cell. Psora spends its action very largely upon the nervous system and the nerve centres, producing 'functional' disturbances.

In **Sycosis**, there are more 'acute' symptoms which have reference to the mucous membranes and the nerve cells. Sycosis attacks the internal organs, especially the pelvic and sexual organs and causes various inflammations and overgrowth of tissues.

In **Syphilis**, symptoms have almost exclusively reference to the nerve cell. Its action is on the cerebral membranes of the brain, and affects the eyes, larynx, throat, bones and periosteum, causing ulceration and destruction.

> **NB:** 'Sycosis' is not synonymous of 'Gonorrhoea'. Sycosis is the whole energetic disturbance, of which the disease Gonorrhoea is but the material part. Also the same can be said for the miasm 'Syphilis' and the disease 'Syphilis'.

The fact that these miasms were called 'Sycosis' and 'Syphilis' by Hahnemann, pointing to their relationship with the inheritance of venereal diseases, is not coincidental. The venereal origin of these miasms stand firm. Since, all our ancestors directly or indirectly were affected through inheritance by them, most diseases have a poly-miasmatic background.

> **NB:** Hahnemann developed the theory about the miasm from his observations in patients who acquired gonorrhoea during Napoleon's invasion from 1809 to 1814.

An affirmation of the venereal origin of these miasms is proved by the fact that some acupuncture meridians that convey the ancestral energy have their points of application in the perineum, namely at the site of the sexual organs (see the chapter of 'Nosodes'). That's why venereal diseases affect our immune system so profoundly, for example AIDS.

Harris L. Coulter explains in his book 'AIDS and SYPHILIS, the hidden link' the major cause of AIDS is the progressive disabling of the immune system by uncured or partially cured syphilis. The other major cause is the drug treatment used for syphilis (and most other diseases). Modern scientific medicine, seeking 'antibiotic sterilization', has relied on medicines whose ultimate effects impairs the patient's immune system.

> **NB:** Sankaran links AIDS to the leprosy miasm, which is a kind of a compilation of pseudo-psora and syphilis.

Acute diseases

Acute diseases are rapid, morbid processes caused by abnormal states and derangements of the vital force. Such affections usually run their course within a brief period of variable duration (H § 72-73).

Acute diseases can be arranged under two groups:

1. Artificial acute diseases are due to over-exertion, injury, over-indulgence, drugs, exposure, unhygienic living or surroundings.
2. True acute diseases are psoric or epidemic. These acute diseases, are mostly due to infectious or contagious miasms which have a specific course by which mostly fever is induced. They usually lead to full recovery or to death.

Chronic diseases

Chronic diseases originate from an infection with a chronic miasm. These miasms create diseases which develop from apparently trifling or imperceptible beginnings, but then advance little by little to maturity and derange in a dynamic way. If not cured by homeopathy, they will finally undermine health and cause death. (H § 72-81)

Psora

Psora (Itch disease – H) is the oldest and also the basic miasm. It is the first cause of all diseases in human organism. Therefore, is often compared with a thousand headed hydra. (H – § 80 and A-II)

Psora itself gives no physiological change of structure, another miasm must be present also in order to produce a physiological change in the structure or shape of part of an organ (A-I). On the other hand, psora, just like the other miasms, is able to cause pathological changes, for example stasis.

The mental symptoms develop after a long illness or at close of severe acute expressions of that miasm, as in typhoid fever (A-I), the psora gets awakened. The mental symptoms are especially anxiety and fear. Furthermore, psora expresses itself by its longings, cravings, aversions and habits of life. Also, the examination of skin may reveal important information (A-I).

The causes of psora, according to Hahnemann are:

1. Contagion
2. Heredity (psora is the primary manifestation of the primeval sin)

Stages of Psora

Primary stage

Psora is so contagious that one can become infected by merely touching the skin, especially in tender children, or by a handshake, or even by a touch of the garments of the affected one. The disposition of being affected is found in almost everyone and under almost all circumstances (H-CD and A-I).

> **NB:** Hahnemann considered psora as a contagious disease causing first physical disturbances and then the mental manifestations. Nowadays, we know that psora is not a contagious disease, as mentioned above, but is a kind of susceptibility (Kent) which is inherent and stored in our genes. The life time of our chromosomes is determined by the number of cell duplications and the length of their telomeres*.

This susceptibility is related to the immune system on which the majority of illnesses depends.

Psora makes its first appearance in the form of pruritus, (10 to 14 days after the infection) followed by fine vesicular eruptions (A-I). No other symptom is so pathognomonic of psora as a pruritus (A-I). Then these manifestations disappear on their own or by suppression and mostly a condition of latent psora remains. This is a condition in which most of the healthy contented people are and stay for an indefinite period of time if they live a healthy normal life. Hahnemann enumerates 60 symptoms of this latent psora in his 'The Chronic Diseases', fifth volume. These symptoms do not reflect a serious disease, so people with such symptoms are considered as healthy by the regular school.

Secondary stage

This latent slumbering psora can become aroused and come into action by getting over-fatigued, either mentally or physically,

---

*   The role of the telomeres:

Telomeres are structures which are situated at the end of the chromosomes and consist of DNA-sequences which do not code for proteins. Of all the DNA there is 3% coded and 97% is non-coded. Only the coded DNA is responsible for the production of the necessary cell proteins. The coded DNA of a chromosome cannot be copied totally from the first cell duplication on without the help of the telomeres. From the first fission, the cell has already too less chromosome material and would die if not the telomeres would give them a part of their structure. So the telomeres become shorter each time the cell duplicates and are by it the marker of the cell ageing.

by some trifling irregularity of life (for example fear, joy), by a slight mental shock (for example grief), injury or change of weather (H-CD and A-I). Even suppression of the simple pruritus can accelerate its development. This aroused condition is called <u>awakened psora</u>. Then profound changes in the organism take place which result in **a neuralgic pain syndrome**, spasms, convulsions, rheumatism and other diseases (A-I). Hahnemann enumerates about 428, symptoms of this awakened psora in his 'The Chronic Diseases', fifth volume.

These symptoms are the elements and manifestations of psora, the original miasmatic malady which now unfolds into forms of disease, with so many varieties, that they are by no means exhausted by the disease symptoms enumerated in the pathology of the regular school medicine, and erroneously designated them as well-defined, constant and peculiar diseases (H-CD).

Tertiary stage

Finally there is development of **internal stasis** in several organs which is often incurable and which leads to coma or death (A-I).

Sycosis

It is important to know the different stages of the sycotic miasm (fig wart disease – H) in the works of S. Hahnemann, J.T. Kent and J.H. Allen.

Stages of Sycosis (Hahnemann and Allen)

Primary stage

It is a stage of acute gonorrhoea that results from a venereal infection by the Neisseria gonorrhoeae. Hahnemann mentions the appearance of verrucae accuminata at the genitals, often, but not always, followed by an urethral discharge. Allen also mentions of a mild cystitis and slight anaemia.

Secondary stage

It starts when those first manifestations disappear, which occurs more quickly if suppressed. Then, the series of secondary disturbances take place in the organism causing a cyanotic mucous congestion, rheumatic sufferings and internal organ stasis, especially in woman's pelvic region causing inflammation and sterility.

Tertiary stage

After a period of some years the tertiary stage starts, hence it is called the genuine sycosis, which may last the patient's whole life, although very often the disease becomes malignant, like scirrhus in several organs, cystic degeneration, fibrous growths, internal organs stasis, chronic rheumatism and gout conditions. This chronic disease can now also be hereditarily transmitted.

> **NB:** J.H. Allen also enumerates some sycotic symptoms in newborns, such as: ophthalmia neonatorum (A-II), uraemic crystals in the urethra, ears, nose and even rectum and vagina

(A-II), excoriating urine and stool (A-II) and a dry stuffed nose (A-II). When the sniffing disappears cramps in the abdomen start, lasting at least for months (A-II).

Conclusion

Now, the sycotic miasm differs from the miasm known in Hahnemann's time. In Hahnemann's time the sycotic miasm was rare. But one century later, J.H. Allen estimated that amid the population of Chicago especially men were sycotic in some degree, either from the acquired form or by hereditary transmission (A-I). The primary manifestation of the sycotic miasm is of bacterial character.

We know from the investigations of Hahnemann and Allen that the contagion can occur by two ways (with some extrapolations*):

1. Sexual intercourse (and saliva*).
2. Vertical transmission: Transmission via mother through the placental barrier (contamination during labour and breast feeding*).

Now a lot of bacteria and viruses, which correspond to these ways of contamination, cause the same disease symptoms as found in the sycotic miasm. **Chlamydia** and the **Human Papilloma Virus (HPV)**, especially types 6 and 11 cause condylomata and genital warts, and also other viral and bacterial agents can be considered, for example Cytomegalovirus (CMV), Epstein-Barr virus (EBV), Herpes virus (HSV-2), Mycoplasma genitalium* and Ureaplasma urealyticum*. (Among lot of these microbes the DNA is found inside the host cell and the DNA of some of them even gets integrated into the host cellular DNA, like HPV infections.)

So, the expression of the primary gonococcus infection has changed nowadays into a wide range of similar infections as mentioned above.

Syphilis

It is important to study the different stages of the syphilitic miasm (the venereal chancre disease–H) in the works of S. Hahnemann, J.T. Kent and J.H. Allen.

Stages of Syphilis

Primary stage

The primary stage is like acute syphilis that results from venereal infection by Treponema pallidum. The period of incubation may vary from 7 to 14 (or even 90) days. It exhibits itself in the form of a chancre. The typical chancre is a solitary, indurated, painless ulcer on or near the genitalia, which heals slowly with scar formation. It is often accompanied by painless enlargement of the regional lymph nodes, the satellite bubo (H-CD and A-I). Hahnemann says that he never had seen an evolution to the following stage if the chancre remains untouched at its place (H-CD). But when a suppression of this vicarious occurs, this organism cause the internal syphilis and break out (H-CD).

Secondary stage

The secondary stage starts 6 to 8 weeks after the primary expression and lasts upto 1 to 2 years. In this period the manifestations appear on the skin and the mucous membranes of the mouth and genitals.

The cutaneous lesions most often found are papules, maculopapules (roseola on the forehead) and follicular papules. Almost any kind of skin eruption may appear <u>except vesicular</u>. Also, localized areas of alopecia frequently occurs, causing a moth-eaten appearance on the scalp. At the mucous membranes painless, superficial erosions appear, which later get covered with a thin, grayish exudation, known as mucous patches.

The mental symptoms usually appear at the beginning or during the secondary stage, probably due to lesions such as congestion of the meninges (A-I). This chronic disease now can also be hereditarily transmitted.

Then, a <u>latent stage</u> or internal syphilis follows which varies between 3 and 12 years. In this stage there are no clinical signs or symptoms of the infection, though it can produce serious changes in the viscera. Suppression can accelerate the development of the different syphilitic stages (A- II).

Tertiary stage

Tertiary stage is not a true syphilis but a combination of psora and syphilis, and that's why it frequently needs anti-psoric remedies for cure (H-CD and A-II). This stage is mainly destructive for:

i. Skeletal system, resulting in multiple bone and teeth manifestations.
ii. Central nervous system, resulting in neurosyphilis.
iii. Cardiovascular system, resulting in cardiovascular syphilis: aortitis with destruction of the media and dilatation of the base of the aorta with regurgitation.

Typical lesions of this stage are the gummas. The gummas begin as painless, subcutaneous tumours that gradually soften and rupture exuding a viscous gummy material.

Conclusion

At present the syphilitic miasm differs from the miasm known in Hahnemann's time. The primary manifestation of the syphilitic miasm is of bacterial character.

We know from the investigations of Hahnemann and Allen that the contagion can occur by two ways (with some extrapolations*):

1. Sexual intercourse (and saliva*).

2. Vertical transmission: Transmission via the mother through the placental barrier (contamination during labour and breast feeding*).

Now a lot of bacteria and viruses, which correspond to these ways of contamination, cause the same disease symptoms as found in the syphilitic miasm. The main amongst them is **the AIDS virus**, but also other viral and bacterial agents can be considered, for example Human Papilloma virus (HPV), especially types 16 and 18 which causes cervical dysplasia and adenocarcinoma, Hepatitis B virus (HBV), Hepatitis C virus (HCV) and Human T-Cell Leukaemia virus (HTLV-1 and HTLV-2). HTLV-1 and HTLV-2 can cause cancer. They are essentially exogenously acquired to the fact that its pro-viral DNA is found only in malignant lymphoma cells. They mainly affect CD4 T-cells and are able to induce malignant transformation in them. They cause adult T-Cell Leukaemia-Lymphoma.

So, the expression of the primary Treponema pallidum infection has changed nowadays into a wide range of similar infections as mentioned above.

Mixed miasm/diathesis

A mixed miasm comes into existence when a **suppression** (by allopathic drugs, radiation, baths, etc.) takes place in an organism when two or more miasms are already present, these miasms get perfectly combined especially by **hereditary transmission**. Through heredity a perfect bond of these miams is formed with the life forces (A-I).

Allen mentions that the more multiple the origin of the mixed miasm is, the more multiple and complex the disease will be, which is originating from that mixed miasm.

Malignancy develops from the mixed miasm, such as cancer lupus, burrowing abscesses, sinuses, tubercular infiltration, growths and all other forms of malignancies (A-II).

Examples of mixed miasm (according to J.H. Allen)

1. Tri-miasmatic (Psora + Sycosis + Syphilis):
    i. The secondary inflammation of sycosis occurs when psora and pseudo-psora blend completely with the sycotic element in the secondary stage (A-II).
    ii. Diseases such as:
        a. Appendicitis (Sycosis + Pseudo-psora) (A-I and A-II).
        b. Cancer, epithelioma (A-I and A-II).
        c. Eczema fissum (Pseudo-psora and Sycosis).
        d. Eczema exfoliata (Psora + Sycosis + Syphilis).
        e. Elephantiasis caused by Tinea.
        f. Lupus vulgaris and erythematosis (Pseudo-psora + Sycosis).
        g. Naevus.

2. Bi-miasmatic:
   i. Psora + Syphilis: Tertiary syphilis (A-II), Pseudo-psora.
   ii. Psora + Sycosis: Alopecia circumscripta, eruptions of vaccination, psoriasis, tinea sycosis / tonsurans / vesicular, verrucae (A-I).
   iii. Pseudo-psora + Sycosis: Worst form of dysmenorrhoea (A-II).
   iv. Sycosis + Syphilis: Condylomata (A-I, A-II).[1]

According to R. Sankaran
1. Tri-miasmatic
   i. Leprosy miasm: Pseudo-psora + Syphilis.
2. Bi-miasmatic
   i. Typhoid (subacute) miasm: Acute miasm + Psora.
   ii. Malaria miasm: Acute miasm in alternation with the sycotic miasm.
   iii. Ringworm miasm: Psora + Sycosis.

---

1. Remedies which are indicated in syco-syphilitic individuals are: asaf., cinnb., merc., nit-ac. and thuj. (A-II).

Tubercular Diathesis

J.H. Allen (1910) added the pseudo-psora or tubercular diathesis to the three classic miasms, which is a combination of psora and syphilis, especially if these miasms are combined by hereditary transmission (A-I).

> **NB:** Pseudo-psora or tubercular diathesis is not synonymous with tuberculosis. The tubercular diathesis is the whole energetic disturbance, of which the disease tuberculosis is but the material part.

Tubercular diathesis causes (A-I):

1. Strong tendency to pustulation or formation of pustules (A-I).
2. Specific, malignant, acute, febrile or inflammatory states, such as pneumonia or diphtheria.
3. Malignancy
4. Syphilis
5. Erysipelas phlegmonous
6. Inflammation of the brain, heart and kidney
7. Destructive appendicitis

Present day picture of the tubercular diathesis is as follows:

1. Antecedents: Open fontanelles, irregular dentition, whooping cough, recurrent colds and bronchitis, pleuritis, primary tuberculosis, adenopathies in childhood, fever of unknown origin, too quick growth, late puberty, chilblains of hands and feet, Raynaud's diseaese, BCG vaccination, etc.
2. Nervous, over-sensitive, extreme lack of energy, need of light and fresh air.
3. <u>Extreme variability of symptoms</u>.
4. Peripheral venous congestion, red cheeks, hypotension, acrocyanosis (which creates a craving for fresh air).
5. Tendency to recurrent febrile attacks. The resisting power of

the immune system is insufficient and it is only by getting fever, which accelerates the basal metabolism and an increased catabolism, that infection can be conquered.
6. Tendency to pustulation or formation of pustules.
7. Elimination occurs through:
   i. Mucosa: Coryza, leucorrhoea.
   ii. Serous membrane: Pleurae, meninges, peritoneum, appendix, etc.
8. Demineralization due to which dehydration, decalcification and fluctuations of the electrolytes occur.
9. Endocrine disturbances: Hyperthyroidism and adrenal insufficiency.
10. Emaciation
11. Chilliness and constipation.
12. Aggravation at night.
13. Target organs: Circulatory system (arterial and venous), lymphatic ganglia and lung.

Scrofulous diathesis

Scrofula[2] is a constitutional state occurring in the young age, marked by lack of resisting power of the tissues predisposing to tuberculosis. There is a tendency to eczematous eruptions, glandular swelling, respiratory catarrh and granular lids. Tuberculosis of glands, bones and joints are common (Sirker, K.K., A Handbook of Repertory).

NB: R.S. Phatak called scrofula as the psora of childhood.

About thousand years ago, scrofula was a plague-like epidemic disease, due to which thousands of people died. The disease was characterized by glandular swelling, especially at the throat, which contained worms. Through generations the disease has lost its plague-like fatal character yet it spread over the West (Lencinus, M., Semper [Belgian medical journal], 1993).

Allen did not make a specific distinction between the tubercular and scrofulous diathesis. The only difference, he said, was in the degree of psoric and tubercular combination, with the conditions of climate, race and other similar associations (A-I). He used an analogy to express the difference: '*As scrofula is the full-grown tree with its luxuriant foliage, tuberculosis is the blossom, often the degenerative stage of scrofula*'.

The development of the scrofulous diathesis is not only due to syphilis and psora combined, but also due to the suppressive measures and crude drugging used in the treatment of syphilis in allopathy. However, there is a remarkable predominance of the syphilitic miasm (A-I).

---

2. Scrofula originated from the latin word 'scrofa' which means swine, because it was known that the fattening pigs used to become the subject to that disease easily.

Miasms

In scrofula there is predisposition to tuberculosis, by which scrofula usually ends in tuberculosis (A-I). Scrofula resembles very much the syphilis diathesis. So their common features are (A-I):

1. Involvement of the lymphatics.
2. Impaired nutrition.
3. Caries and destruction of bones, rickets or softening of bones.
4. Tendency to ulceration.
5. Inflammation of the special sense organs: middle ear, eyes, ciliary apparatus (blepharitis, granular lids) and mucous membranes of mouth, nose and lips.
6. Scrofulides at skin (which resembles syphilides).[3]

List of scrofulous remedies (Repertory of Oscar E. Boericke, C.M. Boger and K.K. Sirker):

Aethi-a., aethi-m., aln., alum., ampe-qu., apis, arg-m., ars., ars-i., all aurums, bac., bad., all barytas, bell., brom., bruc. (Maillé), all calcareas, cann-s., caps., carb-an., card-m., caust., chin., cina, cinnb., cist., clem., coch., con., crot-h., diph., dulc., all ferrums, fl-ac., graph., hell., hep., hydr., all iodides, iodof., kali-bi., kreos., lap-a., lyc., mag-m., all mercuries, mez., all natriums (Cl), nit-ac., nux-v., ol-j., petr., ph-ac., phos., pin-s., psor., puls., rhus-t., ruta, samb., scroph-n., all sedums, sil., sil-mar., spig., still., sulph., syph.*, ther., tub., viol-t.

---

3. Inflammation of the lymphatic glands which spread towards the skin and suppurates and forms irregular cicatrices and nodular swellings in the skin (scrofuloderma).

Cancer diathesis

The cancer diathesis is not synonymous with cancer. The cancer diathesis is the whole energetic disturbance from the beginning, in which ultimately the disease 'cancer' becomes the material expression.

It was Vannier[4a], in 1952, who created the cancer diathesis, a tri-miasmatic state.

Vannier noticed three stages of cancer diathesis:

1. Precancerinic stage.
2. Stage of increasing intoxication which is noticed clinically by brown and black spots on the skin (V-Les cancériniques).
3. Cancerous stage.

Vannier described the cancer diathesis as a miasm of adaptive failure. Vannier made a list of anti-cancer remedies, to be used in the cancerous stage (Vannier - Les cancérniques: see, chapter: Heredity and classic nosodes).

Foubister classified the remedies belonging to the cancer diathesis which belong equally to the Carbonic (Sulphur, Lycopodium clavatum), Phosphoric (Arsenicum album, Natrium muriaticum, Phosphorus) and Sulphuric (Natrium muriaticum, Natrium sulphuricum, Psorinum, Sulphur) constitution of Vannier and Bernard. None of the remedies described by Vannier as fluoric appeared in Foubister's list of related remedies to Carcinosinum.[5]

4a. Vannier, L., Les cancériniques et leur traitement homoeopatiques, Paris : G.Doin & Cie Editeurs, 1952.

L'état cancérinique est l 'ensemble des manifestations objectives et fonctionnelles, locales et générales qui indiquent un terrain cancérinique, un organisme en puissance de cancer.

5. Foubister's list of remedies related to Carcinosinum: alum., ars., ars-i., calc., calc-p., dios., lyc., med., nat-m., nat-s., nux-v., op., psor., puls., sep., staph., sulph. syph., tub.

Features of cancer diathesis

1. Emptiness which is filled by idealism or materialism. For example an empty box is predisposed to be filled up by things from the 'outer' world. So, in the cancer diathesis we see idealistic as well as materialistic people.

   In real cancer, there is a tendency to anaerobiosis, as if being under the ground.[6] So, people of cancer diathesis easily let themselves be dictated by others or become subject to some ideal picture religion or society impose on them. On the other hand they cannot detach themselves from the materialistic world.

2. People having wrong aspirations or deformed, negative or suppressed emotions. This is the result of ignorance concerning the good handling of the emotions. So, this creates a lot of anxiety. Anxiety which finally kills the creativity.

   In the core of this diathesis is the nosode Carcinosinum, which has a fear of frogs. A frog is symbolically related with water and the yin element. The water element stands for anxieties and emotions. In Carcinosinum the anxieties and emotions are suppressed or at least under control.

3. Fear or delusion of having cancer.[4b]

   Children absorb everything from the surroundings like a sponge, so they are addicted to television, computer and read books all the time. They skip their puberty and act directly 'like adults', having an exaggerated sense of duty.

---

6. Cancer cells cannot live in a properly oxygenated body. Normal cells live in aerobiosis. Tumours live in the body almost anaerobically, though on the other hand young metastases live in the body almost aerobically. To prevent cancer it is therefore proposed first to keep the speed of the blood stream so high that the venous blood still contains sufficient oxygen.

4b. Vannier, L., Les cancériniques et leur traitement homoeopatiques, Paris : G.Doin & Cie Editeurs, 1952.

4. Diagonal and cross-wise laterality, e.g. being right-handed and left-footed, or left-handed and right-footed (Pladys, A.).
5. Waking at 4 a.m.
6. Chronic acidification of the connective tissue, which consists of mesenchyma and collagen tissue and is situated around the soft organs, with tendency to alkalosis of the blood (Vincent).
7. Desire sour.
8. Obesity.
9. Metabolic syndrome (with its hyperactivity of the sympathetic nervous system that induces a tissue acidification).

Clinical features of cancer diathesis

1. Ageing, fast [4c].
2. Asthenia, increasing [4b].
3. Physionomy [4d]: Marc Auliffe (1926) noticed that cancer appears more frequently in people of round digestive type and in flat hunchbacked people. Pende noticed it also in people of hyperpituitary type.

    In iridology one notices large but sharp bordered toxic spots of yellowish- brown and red colour at the iris. This is a sign of hereditary predisposition to cancer. In the syphilitic diathesis one finds the same spots but they are smaller.

> **NB:** Vannier thought that the cancer diathesis is only hereditary, and not the fact of certainly getting cancer [4e].

4b. Vannier, L., Les cancériniques et leur traitement homoeopatiques, Paris : G.Doin & Cie Editeurs, 1952.

4c. Vannier, L., Les cancériniques et leur traitement homoeopatiques, Paris : G.Doin & Cie Editeurs, 1952.

4d. Vannier, L., Les cancériniques et leur traitement homoeopatiques, Paris : G.Doin & Cie Editeurs, 1952.

4e. Vannier, L., Les cancériniques et leur traitement homoeopatiques, Paris : G.Doin & Cie Editeurs, 1952.

4. Vannier[4f] also mentions pain on pressure at the second intercostal space, parasternal, bilaterally. According to my experience, these spots are not typical for the cancer diathesis but are rather in relation with a Lycopodium clavatum condition and thus relate to liver intoxication.

BOWEL NOSODES AND MIASMS

Dr John Paterson considered the Bacillus coli as the basic organism from which by the process of mutation, the members of the Bach group (non-lactose fermenting bacilli) originated, thence through the enterococcal stage - the Sycotic co. of Paterson - to the virus.

So, B. coli is the basic organism from which non-lactose fermenting 'bacilli' and 'cocci' originate.

(Source: Lecture presentation showing the technique in the preparation of the non-lactose fermenting nosodes of the bowel and the clinical indications for their use – Dr John Paterson: THE BOWEL NOSODES.)

(Delivered at the 11th Congress of Liga Homoeopathica Internationalis, held in Glasgow, 24th-29th August, 1936. Reprinted from 'The British Homoeopathic Journal, Vol. XL, No. 3. - July 1950. *Published by:* A. Nelson & Company LTD. 73 Duke street Grosvenor Square, London Wim 6BY pg. 214 – 244, quoted parts on p. 234 & 239.)

The Homeopathic Herald: Disease (D. K. Sarkar) :

In the case of what we may call secondary acute exacerbations of the chronic miasmatic illness the internal hypersensitivity is the pertinent factor; only a constitutional treatment can be of real

---

4f. Vannier, L., Les cancériniques et leur traitement homoeopatiques, Paris : G.Doin & Cie Editeurs, 1952.

help. Thus, the term 'miasm' can be taken in the sense of a sum total of all the factors (exogenous and endogenous, psychological, biological and chemicophysical, etc.) in the production of diseased conditions, of which the living microorganisms factor can, of course, never be excluded in case of many acute or chronic diseases. In corroboration of these ideas we may conclude this discussion with the apt remarks of Sir John Weir, which runs thus: 'The miasm came before the microbe. All the evidence would support the theory that the first imbalance was in the host, that the patient suffered form a miasm, an unbalance, a disease which allowed for instance, the B. coli to mutate and become a Gonococcus. He would however, also point out that once the mutation has taken place with the formation of a Gonococcus, it must be accepted that the transference of this infection carrying organism to a healthy person could give rise to Gonorrhoea, but even then one must also consider that there is such a thing as a miasm which could favour the growth of Gonococcus. The Pasteur theory of infection is only a part of the much greater and more scientific doctrine of Hahnemann regarding the true relationship between microorganisms and disease or Miasm.'

– The Homeopethic recorder (September Vol LI N° 9):

Presidential address, June 1936 (J. Weir):

Dr John Paterson of Glasgow, carrying on the work of Wheeler, Bach and Dishington, has demonstrated that the bacterial flora of the bowel also adapts itself to the changes that take place in the organism after the administration of potentised drug. By estimating the proportion and variety of non-lactose fermenters in the stool, he was using the Bacillus coli and its capacity of mutation as an indicator of the effect of the homoeopathic remedy.

– Sankaran P., The elements of Homoeopathy:

The normal B. coli in the intestinal tract performs a useful function and is considered a harmless and non-pathogenic saprophyte. Any change in the human host which affects the intestinal mucosa will upset the balance between the host and bacilli and is followed by a change in the habit and biochemistry of the B. coli which may then mutate (i.e. change in character) and become pathogenic. While this alteration in the nature of the bowel flora might be a mere concomitant to the disease condition there is reason to believe that the change in the nature of the B. coli always follows an alteration in the state of the host, so that the conclusion seems inescapable that diseases are caused primarily and fundamentally as/by a disturbance in the patient (or host) and not by the microorganisms, the disturbance or alteration in the nature of the B. coli occurring only as a consequence and as a reaction to the change in the nature of the environment in the host *. Whereas the normal B. coli ferments lactose, it seems to lose this power when it becomes pathogenic. This alteration can be brought about in several ways, such as by diet, by the potentized drug and by the nosode.

According to J. Paterson, there exists an association of Psora with most bacillary forms (dysenteriae, Morgan-Gaertner, Morgan pure, Mutabile and Proteus), Sycosis with most diplococcal forms (Coccal co. and Syctic co.) and of Syphilis and Pseudo-psora with some different forms (Bacillus 7, Bacillus 10 and Bacillus Gaertner).

Our energetic examination shows another classification than Patersons' in relation to the miasmatic background:

1. Psoric : Coccal, Morgan-Gaertner, Proteus
2. Sycotic : Bacillus 10, Morgan-pure, Sycotic co.

3. Syphilitic : Bacillus Gaertner
4. Tubercular : Bacillus 7
5. Cancer : Dysenteriae, Mutabile

One can consider that the correct application of the Bowel nosodes stimulates the immune system and mostly brings an elimination, by preference via the mucous membranes. Their action is very similar to that of the classic nosodes, which mostly act deeper on heredity (see, chapter: Nosodes).

> **NB:** For more information about the Bowel nosodes, see chapter: 'Bowel nosodes'.

Suppression, Energetic Blockage and The Law of Hering

Suppression and energetic blockage

Suppression in most of the cases is **suppression of the natural tendency to eliminate in a natural disease**. It does not cause any energetic blockage but it accelerates the destructive action of the underlying miasm.

As every disease is linked with the miasm, every suppression of any expression of that disease results in some miasmatic repercussions which makes the internal miasmatic disease evolve faster. It results in a progressive harmful effect on the vital organs.

Psora first affects the ectoderm (skin), before it gives rise to congestion and stasis in the mesoderm and endoderm. The skin is the mirror of the human spirit. So, a suppression of the natural, physiological reaction of the skin gives rise to profound pathological deviation.

The other miasms are secondary to psora and they affect the deeper germ layers. Sycosis affects the endoderm (mucosa) and eventually the mesoderm (heart and circulation), syphilis especially affects the ectoderm (nervous system); the tubercular diathesis especially affects the endoderm and finally the mesoderm (lymphatic system) and the cancer diathesis affects all the germ layers.

When the expression of a miasm is suppressed in one of its stages, the miasmatic disturbance evolves faster in a more destructive way (A-I).

Energetic blockage of a person is mostly caused by some traumatic events, e.g. as a result of surgery, a whiplash, an emotional shock, a wrong homeopathic remedy, a wrong acupuncture treatment, drugs, vaccinations, etc. Such a blockage interferes with the natural developing physiological capacity of the person.

Homeopathy is not harmless and a wrong homeopathic remedy can cause a severe blockage. That is why self medication by the patient must be forbidden.

Law of Hering

By correcting the miasmatic disturbance, e.g. by the action of a homeopathic simillimum, the miasmatic disturbance withdraws its destructive energy from the deeper germ layers and the vital organs and the expression of the disease comes back to surface in the reverse order of its installation, which is called the Law of Hering.

WORK PROCEDURE SKELETON

If after the administration of a well chosen remedy, confirmed by my method of energetic testing, there is no marked amelioration or further evolution of the disease (especially in acute infectious diseases), there are mostly four possibilities to consider (in order of frequency):

1. To give a **classic nosode**, namely Carcinocinum, Medorrhinum, Psorinum, Syphilinum or Tuberculinum, which act on a hereditary blockage and after the administration, the case mostly clears up. This means that the former remedy can now fully unfold its action, even without repeating its intake. This is especially indicated in children (see, chapter: Heredity and nosodes).
2. To give a **bowel nosode**. The blockage in a case is usually due to a hereditary factor, but it is more a blockage in the elimination of stored and waste materials. This is more frequently indicated in adults than in children.
3. To give a **complementary remedy**. The former remedy ameliorate the case a little and there is a standstill, so the remedy is no more indicated.
4. To give an **isopathic nosode**. (How to use isopathic nosodes: see, chapter: Isopathic nosodes.)

> NB: To obtain the exact prescription of the remedy or nosode, you can utilize the list of clinical relationships and confirm the remedy with my method of energetic testing.

(See book: Homoeopathic spiral, flower remedies, kingdoms and remedy interactions; Degroote, F., which is the second part of the first edition of 1994 – to be published.)

The first two possibilities and also the last resemble very much to the primary homeopathic aggravation, yet are not, because there is no following amelioration, but only an aggravation. According to Kent (Lectures on Homoeopathic Philosophy - Lecture XXXV, first[7] and fifth[8] observation), it would be an incurable case.

However, because we encounter it also in young people, it can not only be caused by a too weak energetic state e.g. when giving antibiotics for pneumonia after failure of a homeopathic remedy, the patient ameliorates and comes back in a superficially organic good health, though with a suppressed energetic state. When it repeats often, by taking the allopathic medication, then a much deeper miasm is formed with many layers, which can only be treated by a succession of different miasmatic-related homeopathic remedies.

---

7. First observation: When after administration of a well chosen homeopathic remedy to a patient who is seriously ill and the patient reacts by having a prolonged aggravation which is finally followed by the decline of the patient, the conclusion is that the case was incurable. This failure is due to the impossibility of the vital force to react.

8. Fifth observation: When after administration of a well chosen homeopathic remedy to a patient who is seriously ill, the patient reacts by having first an amelioration followed by a prolonged aggravation, the conclusion is that either the remedy was only superficial and could only act as a palliative, or the remedy was deep and shows that the patient is incurable.

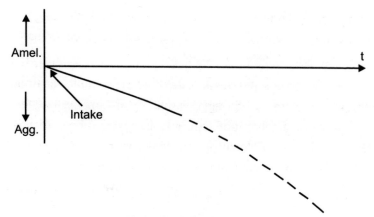

Fig. 1.1 : Kent's First observation

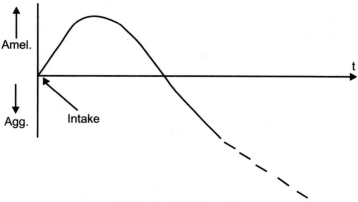

Fig. 1.2 : Kent's Fifth observation

CASES (ILLUSTRATIONS)

Sulphur follows well Allium cepa

A man, 40 years of age, was treated for prostatic troubles with Allium cepa MK by which he reacted well. Six months later, he consulted me again for aching in larynx. The pain ameliorated by eating sweet things and aggravated by warm drinks.

Repertorisation

In the repertory I found: 'Throat, pain, sweet amel.' : Arsenicum album. The burning pain which the patient experienced in the throat corresponded to Arsenicum album, but he appeared to be warm-blooded and his sore throat was aggravated by warm drinks. Moreover, Arsenicum album is not a complementary or satellite remedy of Allium cepa.

In similar case, Dr Pladys extended the rubric to: 'Throat, pain, sweet amel.' and Cough, sugar/sweet/sweetmeats amel.: Psilocybe caerulescens, Spongia tosta, Sulphur. Because Sulphur is warm-blooded and is complementary to Allium cepa, so it was the first to be considered. Our clinical and energetic examination confirmed that option, and Sulphur was given with an excellent result. (A differential diagnosis with Arsenicum iodatum was made as well).

An acute case followed by a nosode

A father consulted me for his daughter of five years, who had a period of fever two weeks before, and after that she had developed cough. The cough sounded loose at daytime, but dry at night. Every time she blew the nose, she had an earache (left). When she had fever, she also had cold feet.

Concerning her mentals, the father told me, she was go-getter, she was really obstinate in getting the desired things. She was afraid in the dark and consequently needed a little light in the sleeping-room. She used to eat in a special manner. Mostly, she ate only one single part of the meal at a time, for example, only the vegetables and not the meat and potatoes. The other time only the meat, and so on.

Repertorisation

1. Cold feet during fever.
2. Loose cough at daytime, dry at night.
3. Ear pain on blowing the nose.

The other symptoms were not taken into consideration for repertorisation because they contained some classic nosodes.

The remedy that was prescribed as a result of the repertorisation was Calcarea carbonica and was indeed also confirmed by the energetic examination. She got a dose of MK.

Follow-up

Four days later, they returned as there was no relief in the child. The child did not like to play alone and had a very changeable humour. Often she cried, and shortly afterwards she laughed again when consoled. Once, when she was not getting what she wanted from the father, she hit his face and broke his spectacles.

Because Calcarea carbonica was well-indicated but did not act, it was indicated to look for a nosode. The changeable mood, the inclination to strike, as an expression of destructiveness, made me think about Tuberculinum. The energetic examination pointed to select Tuberculinum Marmoreck 200K. By this, the hereditary obstruction was taken away and in a few days the girl regained a perfect health.

Nux vomica followed by Syphilinum

An unmarried woman of 39 years old, who consulted me from time to time, has the following sufferings, chronic fatigue with yawning, a bad sleep with frequent waking, unrefreshed feeling in the morning, flatulence, sun allergy and painful rhizarthrosis on the right side. She always had difficulty to recover from a bad or too short night. The last week she dreamt about her dead grandmother in her house and of the furniture which belonged to her. Another dream was concerned about the renovation of a house.

During the clinical examination and observation, I noticed that she had red ears, yet they were cold to touch. The last time I saw her two years ago. She received twice Calcarea fluorica on which she reacted well. I prescribed her Nux vomica MK.

The repertorisation was as follows

1. Ear, discoloration red, yet cold to touch: acon., ail., aloe, ambr., ant-c., apis, ars., bacls-7, bamb-a., bapt. (K), bell., bor-ac., bry., calc-ar., calc., calc-caust., calc-i., calc-p., caps., carb-an., caust., cench., cham., chel., cinnb., con., cor-r., croc., crot-h., dros., equis-h., fl-ac., grat., hep., ip., lac-c., lach., laur., lec., led., lil-t., lyc., mag-c., mag-m., mag-s., med., meph., merc-viv., morg-g., naja-n., nat-m., nat-n. (K), nat-p., nit-ac., nitro-o., nux-v., op., ped., phos., phos-ti., phyt., plat., plb., psor., ptel., puls., rhus-t., rumx., sang., sanic., sep., sil., spig., stram., sul-ac., sul-i., sulph., tab., tarent., tarent-c., verat., vip., vip-t.
2. Loss of sleep aggravates.
3. Rhizarthrosis: am-m., ancls-p., calc., naja, nat-c., NUX-V., rhus-t., sulph., thuj.

Follow-up

A month later she returned. The pain in her thumb had disappeared totally in the first two weeks. Also, she felt more vital. But afterwards her complaints returned partially and that's why she consulted me again.

Again, I noticed the red, cold ears. She complained of a burning pain at the lateral side of hip, extending laterally and downward.

Furthermore, at the shinbone, she had the sensation as if the skin was very vulnerable and was drawn inward into the bone. The sensitivity of the shinbone is a typical of anti-syphilitic remedies.

The energetic examination pointed that Syphilinum MK was prescribed. One month later she called me to tell that everything disappeared very soon after taking the last remedy, and that she was doing fine now.

Staphysagria followed by Medorrhinum

A man of 41 years old, consulted me in June for fistula ani, from which he was suffering for a year. He had already undergone surgery thrice in an university hospital, without any relief. Another complaint was hay fever since he was 18 years old, which was troubling him at that moment.

In his personal anamnesis, at the age of 20, he had a mental breakdown after a disappointment in love. As a child he was easily affected emotionally and he was rather reckless in his playing. He always used to get anxious before an examination and even had some diarrhea. Till he was 30 years old he joined scouting.

For 20 years he was a teacher, a profession which he loved, but he was involved time to time in an open conflict with one of his superior. He could not sustain that this person, who was politically pushed at that place and did not have the required qualities, could dictate him. He was very indignant about that. Therefore, last year, he participated in an examination to get a better job and was selected among many other candidates. Now, he enjoyed his new work, he is obliged to stay at home and had fear to lose this new job because of his illness. This job gave him more esteem and was better paid.

Normally, he was rather impatient and irritable. When angry, he used to shriek, strike, kick and even throw things away. He was extrovert, avoided too bright light, loved rainy weather and practiced judo. He had much fantasy to narrate stories and to write. He was sensitive to clothing, especially around the external throat. Sometimes he experienced difficulty to urinate in the presence of others. During the examination, his jaws cracked when he opened the mouth widely.

Prescription and follow-up

Staphysagria was prescribed and 2 weeks later I saw him back because of an acute lumbago from lifting. The pain was worse on stooping and better while standing and lying. He told that the effect of the dose he took was striking. In one day his coryza stopped and he felt very well. He also went to the surgeon and for the first time there was an improvement in his fistula ani.

The energetic examination pointed Medorrhinum MK for his present illness to be prescribed (according to Dr Pladys, Medorrhinum cures 50 percent of the cases of lumbago and sciatica, and resembles Rhus toxicodendron). His backache disappeared in a few hours and a month later he was totally cured.

Lycopodium clavatum case, who does not react further by Lycopodium clavatum, and needs a nosode to unblock this stagnation

Simon, a four years old boy, was reacting very well by Lycopodium clavatum for two years. But a few months ago he had an otitis on the left side, which did not respond to that remedy anymore.

Yet, he still showed some typical characteristic features of Lycopodium clavatum He was rather egoistic and had a difficult, dominating personality. He was also greedy, often afraid to get too less food. Furthermore, he used to weep at the least trifle, stammered when he is emotional and easily felt overlooked.

Prescription and follow-up

The prescription of a nosode seemed to be indicated here and the energetic examination pointed to Morgan-gaertner (paterson), which is complementary to Lycopodium clavatum. This remedy finally improved his behaviour.

CONCLUSION

What happens after the administration of a well chosen remedy:

1. The stronger the vital force of a patient, who starts a homeopathic treatment, the more the well chosen constitutional remedy can resolve the problem of that patient.

    However, when during the course of that treatment a supplementary acute illness occurs, then the stronger the acute layer, the more there will be a need of an 'acute' remedy (nosodal or / and another) to take away that acute layer.

    This may even happen in people with a strong vital force. Mostly, shortly after treatment of the acute layer, the constitutional remedy must be re-administered.

    Remark: Summer season has a beneficial effect on the vital force of the patient, and vice versa.

2. The less strong the vital force of a patient, the more the well chosen constitutional remedy needs the help of intermediary remedies (nosodal or other remedies) to take away some layers.

So, it happens that, when a well chosen remedy fails, it can be due to a blockage, mostly of an ancestral energy which can be treated by a nosode. In such a case the constitutional remedy can then have a better beneficial effect, when this remedy is prescribed or repeated after the administration of the correct nosode.

So, it is clear that practicing homeopathy without the availability of the nosodes would be rather almost impossible and patients would stay incurable.

Chapter 2

Miasms and their Psychological Background

MIASMS SEEN FROM PSYCHOLOGICAL PERSPECTIVE

In accordance to Sigmund Freud

Psora can be considered as a result of the conflict between the ego and the superego of the individual.

In Freud's last work 'The Ego and the Id' (1923), Freud lined out a new theory of the ego. He showed when the ego and the superego are in constant tension, it often gives rise to morbid mental attitudes, e.g. inferiority complexes, guilt feelings, etc.

Freud considered the psoric miasm as 'Neurosis', (Paschero). Neurosis is a mental disorder without provable neurological or organic dysfunction. It is a light psychological disorder, which burdens the subject and which is experienced as strange, but which does not affect the sense of reality and the social functioning.

Unconscious conflicts create anxieties in the subject by which defense mechanisms are put into action and then cause those dysfunctions.

> **NB:** Hahnemann considered psora as a contagious disease, causing first physical disturbances and in the second place causes mental disturbances. So, we can understand from Hahnemann's point of view that babies can have only skin problems without the mental manifestations of psora.

Paschero incorporated the psycho-analytic conceptions of Freud. So, he considered the disturbed 'morbid' instincts of each person as the 'normal' state and his prescription was based on symptoms originating from those disturbed instinct and feeling. So, what Paschero considered as psora is, according to the insights of Masi, just the result of the suppression of sycosis and syphilis (according to Masi, instincts are morbid).

In accordance to Carl Gustav Jung

The miasm theory of Hahnemann is much in common with Jung's concept of the collective unconscious.

Hahnemann ascertained that the inner state of the subject creates the outer state of that subject and as miasms are strongly related to that inner state and the psyche, they deal with an underlying and collective condition of humanity. So, miasms can be considered as archetypes in the terms of C.G. Jung.

Psora as an archetype

Psora must be considered as an archetype because it corresponds to the definition of an archetype, namely, being a motif that is present in the whole mankind and not only in an individual.

Moreover, psora exists from the beginning of mankind as a hereditary miasm and is symbolically expressed by the 'original sin'. **Psora is a dynamic 'changing' force** linked to the conflict between the self with its collective unconscious and the superego inside the person. So, **Psora acts like a handbrake on the self**, of which it is a part, and consequently slows down and disturbs the individuation process.

Even while treating a patient in a correct homeopathic way, psora cannot be eliminated, which can be understood by the words of Hahnemann who considered psora as a thousand headed hydra.

So, the psora of the patient changes in a dynamic way and comes in contact with other layers of the collective unconscious. This modifies the patient so that a following homeopathic prescription, which can be different of the previous one, is needed.

Features of the psora archetype

1. Want, having:
    i. Original sin, mortality, absence of hereafter
    ii. Insecurity
    iii. Poverty
    iv. Lack of warmth / chilliness
    v. Delusion of being separated, there is no sun behind the clouds
2. Fear of failure
3. Despair of recovery
4. Stasis, mortality

Psorinum is the drug to 'stay alive'. The repeated intake of Psorinum prevents some excessive combustion as well as the falling of life energy.

Psora also corresponds to the 'persona'[1], the mask which counterbalances the personal shadow and the hiding part inside us (relating to the hidden night-side of Dr Jekyll, namely Mr.

---

1. Persona stands for how somebody appears in public, how he is developing, (cf. the ascendant in astrology)

Hyde) and which gives origin to the specific personality traits of each of us.

<u>The other miasms, especially sycosis and syphilis, are linked to the archetypes of especially</u> **the Shadow and that of the Anima/ Animus**.

The other miasms and diatheses must also be considered as archetypes because, they started as an 'individual' infection, having invaded the descendants (family) in a hereditary way they have finally spread themselves in mankind.

This can be compared with the growth of the personal shadow[2] of an individual into the collective shadow of a group. Also, the archetype Anima/Animus[3] is involved in the way, how

---

(Referring to the novel of Stevenson R.L.: The strange case of Dr. Jekyll and Mr. Hyde: Here Dr. Jekyll, a friendly, polite and decent personality, stands for the persona, hiding behind his fiendly mask the secret night-side of Mr. Hyde, who is allowed to show all those emotions regarded as negative: rage, jealousy, shame, greed, avarice, lust, desire to kill.)

Harry van der Zee in his book 'Miasms in labour' shows a correspondence between psora and persona; sycosis and shadow, exploring the unconscious; and between syphilis and anima/animus, magna mater and wise old man.

2. The personal shadow is the negative part in the unconscious of an individual. The ego tends to reject and suppress everything which is experienced as inferior, so that this negative part becomes unconscious. Then the mechanism of projection starts. The negative part is seen in the outer world, as it does not exist any longer inside the subject.

    This corresponds to Freud's unconscious. The collective shadow is the way how a group unconsciously undergoes and acts against feelings of hostility they unconsciously project on the outer world.

3. The anima and animus, or syzygy, constitute an archetype of duality because it is the inner and opposite sex of the individual. The anima is the inner feminine side of a man, and the animus is the inner masculine side of a woman. The anima / animus can be compared to the soul and functions like the unconscious mind. When the projection of anima/animus overrides the conscious will of the individual, the force of the complex dominates the person, as if the person is possessed (Cicchetti, J.: Dreams, Symbols & Homoeopathy, North Atlantic Books).

the psyche and the body physically develop by the influence of the environment, especially in environmental pollution (e.g. increase of oestrogens in the water influences the anima/animus balance), and how the psyche develops by the influence of parental, social and religious education.

These miasms were not heritable primarily yet became heritable by suppression. They also hinder the individuation process[4]. In contrast with psora, these miasms can be treated and eliminated homeopathically (especially by use of classic and bowel nosodes), if necessary over generations. So, a correct homeopathic treatment seems to act in the opposite direction of acquiring those miasms or diatheses.

Especially since the last millennium these miasms are coming more and more into action and are determining our behaviour and the evolution of our society, which nowadays is made up of materialism, imperialism, egotism, travelling, polished apple attitude and moral decay.

Shadow symptoms are often projected onto others. To reveal the Shadow, the following questions can be asked to the patient:

1. Is there anyone whom you strongly dislike and easily get into arguments with?

---

4. The Self is the central archetype that influences all of the archetypal energies with the purpose of moving an individual towards unity, that Jung called individuation. The Self, which encloses both conscious and unconscious, goes beyond and cannot be contained by the individual (Cicchetti, J.: Dreams, Symbols & Homoeopathy, North Atlantic Books).

    The individuation process is a ripening process, which consists of pre-conscious processes, originating from the conflict between the (growing) conscious and the unconscious. These pre-conscious processes come into mind and express themselves in fantasies or in (symbolic) dreams. Individuation also results in being creative.

    (Oerbeelden, De kleine Jung-bibliotheek, Rotterdam: Lemniscaat 2001: Bewust en onbewust, De kleine Jung-bibliotheek, Rotterdam: Lemniscaat 2001).

2. What do you dislike in this person?
3. Which qualities or modes of behaviour do you dislike most in other people?

Answers on these questions can be: e.g. in a Nux vomica patient:

1. People who are aggressive and impolite.
2. People who talk permanently about themselves and who let not others talk.
3. Boasters
4. Liars, people who do not tell the truth.
5. Dictatorial people.
6. Avarice people.
7. Egoistic people.

(Ossege, H.; Homoeopathic Links, vol. 18, 2/05)

For animus/anima, the remedy Sepia officinalis is the example :

Some Sepia-women look mannish, behave more like males and develop a career and they try very hard to be the best mother or housewife.

So, we find in Sepia officinalis an <u>inner split</u> concerning identity. Sepia officinalis has a lack of self-confidence in the ability to become a real wife and mother. So, she struggles continuously with the inner question: Am I a real woman or not.?

The acute miasm corresponds to self-realization. Acute diseases due to natural causes have a specific course during which mostly fever is induced. If one let these illnesses take their course, it will lead mostly to full recovery or to death. (H § 73). For example many people confirm that after an acute disease one make a big jump forward in personal growth. Especially parents have had this experience when their kids pass a childhood disease. That is why childhood diseases are important and vaccinations must be avoided during childhood.

Cancer diathesis

The mean feature of the cancer diathesis is Emptiness (of the individual) by which the person is predisposed to idealism or materialism. For example an empty box is predisposed to be filled up by things from the 'outer' world. So, in the cancer diathesis we see idealistic as well as materialistic people.

These are the two aspects of the same archetype. The positive aspect is related with the mythical motif of the crucifixion, which is a syphilitic feature. It can be recognized in its extremes as an idealism and the tendency to efface oneself.

Otherwise the cancer diathesis is also related with the Anima/Animus archetype, where there is an influence of parental control, religion and education in its largest sense. In the cancer diathesis there is an opposite tendency of self-realization.

An illustration of this is the Dr Coley's famous fever (1870). Dr Coley of New York found that infection is the key to cure cancer. In 1891 he injected Streptococcus pyogenes into inoperable tumours with metastases, which caused a reactionary fever and by this all tumours disappeared.

So, what happens during the cancer process is the opposite of what happens during the action of an acute miasm, which suggests that in the cancer diathesis there is a lack of self-realization on the psychical level.

Recently, a new scientist, on 2nd November 2002, investigated the work of Dr Coley and found spontaneous regression in cancer cases where there occurred an acute infection as flu, measles, malaria, smallpox, etc.

Tubercular diathesis

The tubercular diathesis is related to the negative aspect of the mythical motif of the crucifixion, which is a syphilitic feature.

This corresponds to the tuberculosis illness where there is an inclination to oxygenation, to be compared with a flower away from the ground.

So, people who are subject to the tubercular diathesis tend to leave the reality and the materialistic world.

(See chapter: Classic nosodes: Common features of the ancestral energy out of balance)

(cf.: Scholten, J.: Oxygenium stands for lost self-esteem, victim role and indifference to possession. The oxygenium person is selfish and not idealistic at all.)

Other psychological approaches

Allen, H.: Psychological drives in the creation of a miasm in the individual: The direction of existence of miasms like sycosis and syphilis is through the mind that man sins and becomes diseased. This is true in most of the cases that diseases emanate from lust. Here we find the typical triune: he thinks, he wills, he acts, and out of that triune comes the visible physical manifestations of the venereal disease.

The mind is the vice-regent of the body, the government, the ruling power. The body is subject to it in many ways and therefore subservient to it. So, if we violate a law of principle of life related to the mind, the body cannot shield it because the body is subjected to the same law (A-I).

Masi Elizalde, A.: Psychological background of miasms: The primary psora is considered as a state of suffering without an explanation i.e. being aware of one's vulnerability, or a feeling of nostalgia, guilt or punishment.

Masi considered the content of the collective unconscious of Jung as the primary psora (Masi, Cours supérieur. He also put forward that the primary psora is located in the imagination (Masi, Cours supérieur.) The other miasms are considered as dynamic reaction on that primary state.

Psora, secondary: Projection of the anxieties to the outer world. This relates to the shadow, which is the negative part of the psyche. People tend to suppress that negative part, so that it becomes unconscious. Then the mechanism of projection starts. The negative part is seen by the outer world, as it does not exist any longer inside the subject.

Reactions on this psoric process, which Masi called the tertiary psora, are:

Sycosis : Hyper-reaction to maintain oneself.

Syphilis : Hypo-reaction or auto and hetero-destructive reactions, when one cannot stand up to some circumstances.

> **NB:** The tubercular and the cancer diatheses do not have its own individuality or personality. (Masi, Cours supérieur)

Sankaran, R.: Miasms are reaction types: Miasms, as Sankaran describes are very different from the classical traditional miasms. His ten (what he calls) miasms express the way of being, of perceiving the world and of handling problems. So, they are a kind of reaction types, which are much like the stages as used in the periodic table of elements.

(See, Homoeopathic Links, vol. 20, and vol. 22)

Miasms and other approaches

1. Miasms and the elements

Together with the seasons and the human temperaments, the four elements complete the doctrine of the correspondence between the macrocosmos and the microcosmos, the believe in analogy between man and universe as a whole.

i. Water (wet/cold) corresponds to winter and the phlegmatic temperament.
ii. Fire (dry/hot) corresponds to summer and the choleric temperament.
iii. Earth (dry/cold) corresponds to autumn and the melancholic temperament.
iv. Air (wet/hot) corresponds to spring and the sanguine temperament.

According to Chaim Rosenthal:

i. Psoric miasm: Earth
ii. Sycotic miasm: Water
iii. Syphilitic miasm: Fire
iv. Tubercular diathesis: Air
v. Cancer diathesis: Fire + Air
vi. Leprosy: Water + Fire
vii. Typhoid: Earth + Air
viii. Ringworm: Earth + Water
ix. Malaria: Water + Air
x. Acute miasm: Fire + Earth

2. Miasms and Tridosha / Ayurveda

The macrocosmos is composed of three elements:

i. Vata (V) corresponds to air (and water), life force (prana), motion, small and large intestines and nervous system. Vata is adapted to nervous and irritable people. Vata is a Sanskrit word that means 'wind' or 'that which moves'.

ii. Pitta (P) corresponds to fire (and water), circulation, gall, the duodenum, inflammation and aggression. Pitta is adapted to fiery people.

iii. Kapha (K) corresponds to water (and earth), coldness, mucous membranes, mucous (phlegm) and phlegmatism. Kapha is adapted to self-controlled people. Kapha means 'that which holds things together'.

Analysis of the work of Benoytosh Bhattacharya led me to the following conclusions:

i. Psoric miasm corresponds especially to Vata and Kapha.
   a. K: Calcarea carbonica.
   b. VK: Psorinum.

ii. Sycotic miasm corresponds especially to Vata and Kapha.
   a. VK: Medorrhinum.
   b. P: Kalium muriaticum.
   c. V: Natrium phosphoricum.
   d. VP: Natrium sulphuricum*, Nitricum acidum, Thuja occidentalis.

iii. Syphilitic miasm corresponds especially to Pitta and Kapha.
   a. K: Aurum metallicum, Fluoricum acidum.
   b. P: Kalium muriaticum, Syphilinum.
   c. PK: Aurum muriaticum natronatum, (all) Mercury remedies.
   d. VK: Arsenicum iodatum, Iodium.

iv. Tubercular diathesis corresponds especially to Vata and Pitta.
   a. K: Drosera rotundifolia.
   b. VP: Bacillinum, Tuberculinum

      c. VK: Arsenicum iodatum, Iodium, Calcarea phosphorica, Kalium phosphoricum, Magnesium phosphoricum.
- v. Cancer diathesis corresponds especially to Pitta and Kapha.
    - a. P: Bromium, Carbo animalis, Ceanothus americanus, Condurango, Sabina.
    - b. K: Scrophularia nodosa.
    - c. PK: Carcinosinum*, Ornithogalum umbellatum.
    - d. VK: Badiaga.
    - e. VP: Nitricum acidum.
    - f. VPK: Ammonium carbonicum, Badiaga., Conium maculatum.
- vi. Leprosy corresponds especially to Pitta and Kapha.
- vii. Typhoid corresponds especially to Vata, Pitta and Kapha.
- viii. Ringworm corresponds especially to Vata and Pitta.
- ix. Malaria corresponds especially to Vata and Pitta.
- x. Acute miasms correspond to Vata, Pitta and Kapha.
    - a. Chicken pox: VK.
    - b. Cholera: VPK.
    - c. Measles: PK.
    - d. Small pox: PK.
    - e. Vaccinia: VPK.

Acute and chronic severe diseases must be treated preferably first with a VPK remedy, of which only eight are known, namely: Ammonium carbonicum, Ammonium muriaticum, Baptisia tinctoria, Camphora officinalis, Crocus sativus, Ferrum metallicum, Ferrum phosphoricum and Sepia officinalis. Thus, V remedies, namely VK, VP and VPK remedies, are the most important, followed by the other remedies.

Chapter 3

Heredity

ANCESTRAL ENERGY

The ancestral energy is the hereditary energy coming from the ancestors. Chromosomes are carrier of the ancestral energy.

The conventional view is that DNA, in its sequence, carries all the hereditary information and even that which individuals do not acquire in their lifetime, it is biologically passed to their children.

DNA is also wrapped in a layer of chromatin proteins which are methylated to the DNA molecules and protect the DNA-helix. So, the negative information present in the DNA can only become active when the chromatin proteins on that place do not protect the DNA anymore (Results from investigations at the University of Gent - 2001 and Brussels - 2006)

So, an aberrant methylation of the DNA plays a primordial role in cancerogenesis. Disorders of the DNA methylation occur in about 65 percent of the cancers. A disturbed methylation leads to an inactivation of the tumour suppressor genes and leads to the development of cancer.

Nowadays, scientists according to epigenetics are researching that hypermethylation of DNA is a key element in the development of cancer.

The idea is that inheritance is not just about which kind of genes one inherits but also which of these are switched on or off is a whole new frontier in biology. It raises questions with huge implication to find what sort of environmental effects can affect these switches. So, the stabilization of the perfect methylation of the chromatin proteins around the DNA is needed to keep the patient in good health.

From the energetic point of view, the stability of those chromatin proteins is influenced by an ancestral energetic layer which can be kept stable by the use of nosodes which are directly related to the ancestral energy.

> **NB**: 3% of the DNA is coded DNA and 97% is non-coded, the so-called junk DNA.
>
> In that junk DNA there are a lot of unstable tandem repeats of pieces of DNA which have an important role in the gene expression because those repeats of pieces of DNA influence the wrapping structure of the DNA by chromatin proteins.(Science, 2009 May 29)
>
> Moreover most of diseases are related to a lot of genes, sometimes even hundreds of genes.

Recent evolution about insights concerning DNA

Now the epigenetic theory adds a whole new layer to genes beyond the DNA. Biology stands on the brink of a shift in the understanding of inheritance. The discovery of epigenetic hidden influences upon the genes would affect every aspect of our life. When examining the genome, scientists discovered that the number of genes were lesser than expected according to the numerous functions. The sequence of the genome is insufficient to understand our diversity and complexity. That's why we have to pay attention also to the chemical reactions around the DNA molecule.

Marcus Pembrey, a Professor of Clinical Genetics at the Institute of Child Health in London, started studying about this because he was fascinated by the paradox that the lack of a part of chromosome 5 causes Prader Willy syndrome when it is inherited from the father and Angelman syndrome when inherited from the mother. So, even when the DNA sequence is the same, the kind of disease depended on it can be inherited from the father or mother.

He concluded that genes have a memory of their origin. His conclusion was that one gene or a lot of genes related to one disease cannot explain everything.

In a remote town in northern Sweden he found an evidence for this radical idea. In Överkalix's parish registry of births and deaths, its detailed harvest records which confounded traditional scientific thinking. In collaboration with Swedish researcher Lars Olov Bygren, found evidence in these records of an environmental effect being passed down the generations. It had shown that a famine at critical times in the lives of the grandparents can affect the life expectancy of their grandchildren. This was the first evidence that an environmental effect can be inherited in humans.

What kind of person's parents and grandparents had lifestyle appeared to have a significant impact on their risk of cardiovascular disease and diabetes, Bygren's team reports in the European Journal of Human Genetics (2002;10:682-688). People whose relatives had lived through a famine with a lower risk of disease, according to the report, for people whose fathers did not have enough food during the 'slow-growth' period of childhood and before puberty, their risk of cardiovascular disease was lower than normal. To a lesser extent, the same was true for people whose paternal grandmother had lived through a famine. Similarly, having a paternal grandfather who had lived through a famine was associated with a lower risk of diabetes. But if a paternal grandfather had plenty of food during his 'slow-growth' period, his grandchildren were about four times more likely to die with diabetes.

The epigenetic effect through the grandmother occurs when the child is still in uterus and through the grandfather it occurs just before puberty, the slow growth period between the ages of 9 and 12.

Environmental factors experienced by a woman during the period of 'the ripening of the egg cell and the resulting pregnancy' and by a man 'during the maturation of the spermatogenesis process before puberty' leave a trace in following generations.

So, epigenetics can be a link between the modern science and the homeopathic miasmatic approach.

If we consider the results of the research until now concerning epigenetics is a kind of 'memory' transmitted through generations. Also, in scientific environment the genetic information no longer seen as something static but as something that is flowing. This idea of 'flowing of the genetic information' corresponds to the concept of miasms in homeopathy. As homeopaths we all know the importance of the familiar antecedents and **the state of the mother during pregnancy** in our analysis.

Mostly, if a classic nosode is indicated, it will be in an intermediate way, for example when the well selected remedies failed. Then, the prescription of the nosode usually is based on the family and personal history. The predominance of nosodal symptoms in babies and infants is usually striking. This means that nosodes are more indicated in childhood as compared to adolescence. Nosodal energy acts especially upon some extra-channels, vessels or meridians, which transport inheritable forces, the ancestral energy. These forces are bound with the chromosomes and they come from our ancestors. So, it is not something particular to the individual but common to a large number of his relatives (epigenetics). The ancestral energy determines the great part our immune system and life force and it also explains the tendencies to several illnesses in the form of so called congenital weakness.

DIAGNOSIS

By kinesiologic testing

This test is executed on a strong indicator muscle, e.g. the musculus deltoideus anterior, serratus anterior or rectus femoris.

There is a general handmode which indicates a miasmatic disturbance to explore the miasmatic field:

1. MD: T2-Ic, IMRL 90 degrees finger flexion (Alan G. Beardall).
2. MD: T3-M4, M extended, IR flexed, OL (Alan G. Beardall).

When a strong indicator muscle tests 'weak' on that MD, it indicates a hereditary weakness, which usually relates to one of the classic nosodes or some miasmatic isopathic agent (see Chapter: Isopathic nosodes).

Then the diathesis, which is substantially disturbed, can be traced as follows:

i. Psora (referring to the crab louse): Both hands alternately crossed above the pubic region.
ii. Sycosis: Legs at ankles alternately crossed.
iii. Syphilis: Forearms alternately crossed in front of the chest.

iv. Tubercular (scrophula): Arms alternately crossed over the navel.

Also by Therapy Localization (TL), the weakest diathesis can be traced:

i. Sycotic diathesis: TL on the right mastoid process.
ii. Syphilitic diathesis: TL on the left mastoid process.
iii. Tubercular diathesis: TL at 2 cm distance (mostly left) from the anterior fontanelle.
iv. Cancer diathesis: TL on the convex line in the middle between the right ear and the caudal extension of the sutura sagittalis under the linea nuchae suprema.

If one of these diatheses is present, there is a positive TL at Conception Vessel 24 **(CV 24, alarm point of the ancestral, hereditary energy)** by which the strong indicator muscle becomes weak.

The lateralization of the 'superposing' member refers to the origin of the weakness :

1. Left: Side of the ovum : Mother.
2. Right: Side of the sperm : Father.

For example when Medorrhinum is indicated and there is a related weakened muscle of which only one of the two lateralities is possible, then the disturbance originates from father's side if the right musculus supraspinatus is weakened, and from the mother's side if the left musculus supraspinatus is weakened.

By anamnesis

I. Family anamnesis

It is important to know the family history of the patient to obtain a wide view over his clinical history. So, it is not only important to go into the family history of the father, mother, sisters and brothers, but sometimes it is of more importance to know the clinical history of uncles and aunts, when considering heredity.

i. **Sycotic state:** Suppressed gonorrhoea, heart diseases, myocardial infarction in young people, hypercholesterolemia, arteriosclerosis, Down's syndrome, pernicious anaemia.

ii. **Syphilitic state:** Suppressed syphilis, heart affections, hereditary tendency to alcoholism, recurrent miscarriages, premature births, high perinatal mortality, children in the same family who do not resemble each other in appearance and height, saddle nose, Hutchinson teeth.

iii. **Tubercular state:** Tuberculosis, neuraesthenic, artistic family, astigmatism.

iv. **Cancer state:** Cancer and leukaemia among near relatives, tuberculosis, congenital hereditary syphilis, pernicious anaemia, diabetes and peptic ulcers.

2. Personal anamnesis

Because of the dominating role of hereditary power in children, childhood is very important in the anamnesis.

i. **Psoric state:** Skin eruptions, **measles**, eczema, parasitic diseases (dd.: Cancer state), obesity, **hypotension**, aggravation in the morning and amelioration in the open air.

ii. **Sycotic state:** Colic-babies, **scarlet fever** (in which there is a peri-anal redness), recurrent coryza, pelvic inflammations, warts, rheumatism, gout, **influenza**, repeated vaccinations, heart and vascular diseases (increased cholesterol), sterility, **mumps**, **endometriosis**, over-sensitiveness to damp weather, dropsy, over-sensitiveness to sea-air (dd.: Cancer state), aggravation during daytime and amelioration at night.

iii. **Syphilitic state:** Premature birth, atrophic placenta, **small-for-date child, scarlet fever**, chicken pox, difficult growth, open fontanelles, blue sclerotics, saddle nose, Hutchinson teeth, **yellow-orange colour of the palate** (sign of Naret), split uvula, irregular implantation of teeth because of lack of space, an oblique eye line with respect to the axis of the face, macrocephaly, backwardness (dd.: Cancer state), psychosis, hereditary alcoholism, hereditary **liver disorders** (i.e. increased gamma-GT and alkaline phosphatase), neurological affections, valvular diseases, **aneurysm of the aorta**, amelioration in the mountains, aggravation at night.

iv. **Tubercular state:** Imperfect teeth in an irregular order with early decay, open fontanelles, hairy growth on face and back in children, long eyelashes, very fine hair, mental precocity, late puberty, baby-face, **red cheeks**, ganglionary adenopathies in children, recurrent colds, bronchitis, **whooping cough**, fever of unknown origin, too quick growth, emaciation, aggravation at night, amelioration in the open air, **hypotension, bright red lips**, Raynaud's disease, chilblains on hands and feet.

v. **Cancer state: Whooping cough** or bad pneumonia usually in the first two years of life, absence of the children illnesses or children illnesses at an older age, coeliac disease, bizarre tics, insomnia, porcelain blue sclerotics, dark circles around the eyes, a pale brownish café-au-lait complexion, earthy discolouration of face, constipation, coeliac disease, increased cholesterol, **arterial hypertensive patients with bright lilac to red violet lips and varicose nose**, or pale lips (never bright red lips), fissures at the labial commissures and fissured tongue, comedone in adults, molluscum pendulum at the cervical region, little red spots on abdomen and thorax whose size varies from pinhead to that of a small pea (yet are not naevi), keratosis senilis, verrucae seborrhoica, warts, papilloma, condylomata, moles, numerous naevi and neurasthenia.

> **NB:** A confusing symptomatology points to several miasms e.g. J.H. Allen and G. Vithoulkas.

TREATMENT

By homeopathy

'**One miasm contains different layers and must consequently be treated depending on the predominating actual miasm'** (S. Hahnemann, J.H. Allen, P.S. Ortega and G. Vithoulkas). This can be done by the different kinds of remedies.

1. Nosodes

The intercurrent administration of especially the classic nosodes (Carcinosinum, Medorrhinum, Syphilinum and Tuberculinum) and the Bowel nosodes give the the quickest and most effective way to treat the herediatry load in a person because each of these nosodes reflect the centre point of the corresponding miasm.

When we have the opportunity to administer the appropriate nosode shortly after the intake of the simillimum for the awakened underlying miasm, then the hereditary binding of that miasm with the vital force will easily be broken up. Yet, there is one exception, namely Psorinum, which refers to the basic miasm psora, which is the thousand headed hydra, and cannot be fully destroyed (H- § 80).

So, the administration of Psorinum must be repeated frequently during the lifetime.

Some hereditary blockages can also be removed by nosodes, originating from **isopathic agents** (for example: AIDS nosode, Chlamydinum, Chlamydinum trachomatis, Herpes genitalis, etc.) because they are very near to corresponding miasm to treat. Sometimes also auto-isopathic agents (for example blood, urine, etc.) can be used.

2. Non-anti-psoric Remedies

By using only those kind of remedies, that unlinking of the miasms, decrease the ageing and degeneration process from the vital force.

i. **Anti-sycotic remedies:** Agar., alum., am-c., aran., arg-m., arg-n., arn., aster., bapt., berb., bry., canth., caps., caust., cham., chin., cimic., clem., colch., coloc., croc., crot-h., crot-t., cub., dulc., gels., hydr., kali-s., lac-c., lach., luna, lyc., mag-c., maland., murx., nat-s., nit-ac., nux-m., nux-v., petr., phyt., puls., pyrog., rhus-t., sars., sep., staph., sulph., ter., thuj., vac.

ii. **Anti-syphilitic remedies:** Anan., arg-n., ars., asaf., aur., aur-m., aur-m-n., bar-c., benz-ac., bism., cinnb., cub., fl-ac. and all fluoric-remedies (calc-f., kali-f., nat-f., nat-sil-f., ...), hydrog-perox.*, iod. and all iodide-remdies (ars-i., aur-i., calc-i., kali-i., merc-i-f., merc-i-r., sul-i., ...), kali-ar., kali-bi., kalm., kreos., led., merc., merc-c., mez., nit-ac., phyt., pilo., plat., podo., thuj.

iii. **Anti-tubercular remedies:** Acet-ac., ars., ail., am-c., am-m., brom., calc., calc-ar., calc-p., (carb-v.), chin., cocc., cupr., dros., elaps, ferr., graph., ham., hep., (all iodide-remedies), kali-c., kali-m., lac-d., lil-t., lob., mag-m., mill., nat-c., nat-m., petr., phos. and all phosphor-remedies (am-p., calc-p., kali-p., mag-p., nat-p., ph-ac., phos., ...), puls., sil., stann., sul-i., ther., viol-o. and zinc.

iv. **Specific Anti-cancer 'palliative' remedies according to Vannier and others :** Am-c.$_{tridosha}$, ars., ars-r., aster., aur-m-n., bad., brom., cadm., calen., calc-ar., carb-ac., carb-an., card-m., cean., cere-b., chel., chin., chim., chol., cholin., cinnb., cinnm., cit-ac., con., cund., euph., form., fuli., gali., ger., helon., hura, hydr., hydr-ac., kali-cy., kali-perm., microc., nit-ac.$_{sk7}$, orni., oscillo., phos., phyt., rad-br., ruta, sabal., sabin., sang., sars., scir., scroph-n., sed-ac., solid., strych-g., thlas., thuj., x-ray.

NB: In the pre-cancerinic state, 'vegetable' remedies are the best to modify the organism gently.

3. Anti-psoric Remedies

Agar., alum., am-c., am-m., ambr., anac., ars., aur., bar-c., bell., borx., bov., bufo, calc., carb-an., carb-v., caust., cer-b., chin., cist., clem., coff., coloc., con., dig., dulc., euph., graph., guaj., hep., ign., iod., kali-c., kali-n., lob., lyc., mag-c., mag-m., mang., merc-d., mez., mosch., mur-ac., nat-c., nat-m., nit-ac., nux-v., orig., petr., ph-ac., phos., plat., psor., rhod., rumx., sal-ac., sars., sep., sil., stann., sulph., zinc.

(Hahnemann: Trait, des maladies chroniques, 3* édition française par P. Schmidt and J. Künzli and Boenninghausen)

Note

Kent writes in Lecture XXII of his 'Lectures on Homoeopathic Philosophy': By writing the remedies related to the disease symptoms of psora, mentioned by Hahnemann in his 'Chronic Diseases'(H-CD), you will find the list of the anti-psoric remedies. Doing the same with sycotic disease symptoms, you will find the list of the anti-sycotic remedies. It is interesting to use the symptoms of sycosis mentioned by S. Hahnemann, J.T. Kent and J.H. Allen. And, doing the same with syphilitic disease symptoms, you will find the list of the anti-syphilitic remedies.

By hygiene

1. Weight control, healthy food and a regular way of life are also required for the treatment.

For example:

i. In tubercular diathesis usually there is a bad nutritional condition of the body. Therefore, a nourishing diet is required, such as raw eggs, raw vegetables and certain fats such as milk, cream, butter and olive oil. (If for a long term, the patient has not consumed milk, its intake should be started again little by little because of the adaptation to digest lactose).

On the other hand, milk should not be given to tubercular children, because it can cause several clinical pictures such as diarrhoea, spasms, convulsions, etc. Children with worms should be forbidden to eat meat and potatoes for a while.

Moreover the tubercular patient needs plenty of fresh air and sunshine, exercise and appropriate bathing. Sleeping with open window is recommended.

ii. The most vulnerable organs of the sycotic patient are the heart and blood vessels. Also, there is often an overfeeding, even intoxication, of the body.

Therefore, it is recommended to have plenty of physical exercise, to take a low-fat and low-protein diet and to avoid alcoholic drinks and allopathic drugs. It is also highly recommended to take hot baths and to drink alkaline mineral water (to improve the kidney function and to buffer the increased amount of uric acid in the blood).

NB: Remark: An increased uric acid level is known as a risk indicator for the heart (hypertension, myocardial infarction) and diabetes. However one must be cautious when taking too much of alkaline water because it can disturb the own production of sodium bicarbonate.

iii. In the cancer and sycotic diathesis, the tissue acidification must be corrected by the higher intake of alkalizing foods, such as potatoes, green vegetables (no garden cress, garden sorrel and rhubarb), milk, yoghurt, cream, bananas, chestnuts, almonds and fruit.

And on the other hand, acidizing food must be reduced, such as animal proteins, meat, fish, butter, cheese, fats and oils, white sugar, peanuts, grains, white flour and its products (like white bread, white pasta, etc.), beans, alcoholic drinks, tea, coffee, etc. Also 'Alfalfa' (= lucerne) 500 mg – Soria Natural (3 x 2 tablets a day), **alkalizing citrates**, carbonates and alkaline antioxidant water are recommended to be taken.

Table I : Alkalizing Foods

Green vegetables	Fruits	Others
Garlic	Apple	Apple cider vinegar
Fermented veggies	Avocado	Bee pollen
Beets	Banana	Lecithin granules
Broccoli	Cantaloupe	Probiotic cultures
Cabbage	Cherries	Green juices
Carrot	Currants	Veggies juices
Cauliflower	Dates/Figs	Fresh fruit juice
Celery	Grapes	Organic milk (unpasteurized)
Chard	Grapefruit	Mineral water
Chlorella	Lime	Alkaline antioxidant water
Collard greens	Honeydew melon	Green tea
Cucumber	Nectarine	Herbal tea
Eggplant	Olives	Dandelion tea
Kale	Orange	Ginseng tea
Kohlrabi	Lemon	Banchi tea
Lettuce	Peach	Kombucha
Mushroom	Pear	
Mustard greens	Pineapple	**Sweeteners**

Green vegetables	Fruits	Others
Dulce	All Berries	Stevia
Dandelions	Tangerine	
Edible flowers	Tomato	**Spices/Seasonings**
Onion	Tropical fruits	Cinnamon
Parsnips (high glycemic)	Watermelon	Curry
		Ginger
Peppers	**Protein**	Mustard
Pumpkin	Egg yolk	Chilli pepper
Rutabaga	Whey protein powder	Sea salt
Sea veggies	Cottage cheese	Miso
Spirulina	Chicken breast	Tamari
Squashes	Cream	All herbs
Alfalfa	Yoghurt	
Barley grass	Almonds	**Oriental vegetables**
Wheat grass	Brasil nuts	Maitake
Wild greens	Chestnuts	Daikon
Nightshade veggies	Tofu (fermented)	Dandelion root
	Flax seeds	Shitake
	Pumpkin seeds	Kombu
	Tempeh (fermented)	Reishi
	Squash seeds	Nori
	Sunflower seeds	Umeboshi
	Millet	Wakame
	Sprouted seeds	Sea veggies

A pre-cancerinic patient must be encouraged to eat beets to stimulate the liver function. Also, the kidney function must be stimulated by drinking large amount of mineral water. A vegetarian diet is recommended and the use of coffee and chocolate must be forbidden. Also sleeping early is necessary.

In a 'cancer' patient there is a tendency to anaerobiosis and also a whole process of cellular intoxication. This causes the outfall of the genome which activates the apoptosis in the cell and deviates it from its normal state. Contrary to the pre-cancerinic state, in cancer patients some spectacular results are obtained by administering DCA (sodium dichloroacetate) in high dose (e.g.: 300 mg, twice a day). The probably good effect of acid had already suggested by the fact that most cancer patients crave sour things, like champagne.

The working mechanism supposes that the high intake of acids changes the pH value inside the cell which deblocks the suppressed apoptosis genome, so that the cancer cell kills itself. Acids also stimulate the liver function and its Kupffer cells which belong to the reticuloendothelial system (Clarke recommends not to give milk and salt to cancer patients).

During the day there is an increasing acidification of the tissues with a compensatory alkalization in the blood. Whereas during the night there is an eliminatory process in the reversed way.

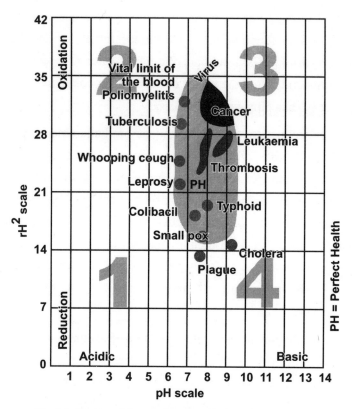

Fig. 3.1 : Health and the most important diseases (the human biological field) (source: http://www.bevincent.com)

In fig. 3.1 we see also a link to the nowadays known homeopathic miasms.

a. The first quadrant which represents an acid-deoxidized environment, which links to the psoric miasm (at right upper corner).

b. The second quadrant represents an acid-oxidized environment, which links to the tubercular, scrofulous, syphilitic, ringworm and lepra diathesis.

c. The third quadrant represents an alkaline-oxidized environment, which links to the sycotic miasm and cancer diathesis. (p-69)
   d. The fourth quadrant, represents an alkaline-deoxidized environment, which links to the acute miasm, malaria, cholera and typhoid diathesis.
2. Diet and fasting cures, e.g. the Mayr therapy.
3. Supplementary nutrients: Minerals, vitamins, oligo-elements, proteins, RNA/DNA,etc.
4. Sport, relaxation, massage, baths, etc.
5. Surrounding factors: Work and relations (stress), living area, etc.

By psychotherapy

The goal is to achieve the balance between oneself and his environment. It is highly important to learn to express and to deal with own emotions. The delusion at the base of the illness has to be elaborated. Once the person appreciates his own delusion this begins to work on him like a homeopathic remedy.

(cf. R. Sankaran: The homeo-psychotherapy: Disease is delusion and awareness is cure.)

By other therapies

For example acupuncture, hydrotherapy, osteo-articular therapy, neural therapy, allopathy,etc.

Chapter 4

Heredity and Classic Nosodes

In homeopathic practice it is sometimes difficult to select the appropriate remedy via classic repertorisation, according to the criteria given by Hahnemann in the 'Organon of Medicine' (§ 95, 98, 209, 99, 84, 18, 26, 153, 164, 165, 209, 210, 213, foot notes 25 and 81, 276, 269, 273, foot note 80) and by Kent (in his 'Lectures', chapters XXX to XXXIV, and in his 'Lesser Writings' or by the dynamic miasmatic concept of the (mental) symptoms as designed by Masi Elizalde, the common remedy that covers 'all' characteristic symptoms. On the contrary, we obtain a few remedies (similae) of which none covers all the totality of symptoms.

What remedy is consequently the simillimum? In some cases by the knowledge of the nuclei the proper remedy can be distinguished easily, but in other cases the choice is not that evident. May be we have to reconsider the anamnesis or the selection of the symptoms, or there are too little proved remedies. May be the symptoms of the corresponding remedies are not sufficiently known (cf. Additions to the repertory of Kent based on the various materia medica as already partially done by C. Boger, H. Barthel, W. Klunker and many others), or may be the symptoms have to be selected in a different way.

Until now, an artifice is used to subdivide the totality of symptoms (concerning the present and the past), through the approach of the chronic miasms, as educated by Hahnemann.

According to Hahnemann (H – § 209 and 'H – CD' - Cure of the chronic diseases, J.H. Allen and P.S. Ortega, first of all the 'active predominated' miasm should be treated.

For instance :

1. When psoric expressions are predominant, then anti-psoric remedy must be administered (also for tertiary syphilis).
2. When sycotic expressions are predominant, first anti-sycotic remedy and afterwards anti-psoric remedy should be given.
3. When syphilitic expressions (in first or second stage) are predominant, then anti-syphilitic remedy should be administered before anti-psoric remedy.

However, by using this method, we cannot conceal that we neglect the totality of the symptoms of one person in a certain way On the other hand, the dynamic miasmatic concept according to A. Masi Elizalde speaks in favour of a more totalitarian approach - to the patient as well as to the remedy, in which the three classic miasms are united and treated by one remedy.

This approach is based on a 'human image', that is the two-parted human image according to Thomas Van Aquino. Man is considered as one indivisible entity composed by a soul and a spirit. So, man, who is a spiritual being, is striving during his lifetime to regain the optimal balance with respect to himself, his environment, the whole Cosmos and God before the fall.

In the anthroposophy, founded by Rudolf Steiner, the personalistic human image is emphasised. This means that next to the inherent heredity factors and surrounding influences, a third power comes to the front and that is the personality or individuality. So, from birth, one signs step by step to his own unique biography.

The human being participates in two different worlds. The first is the earthly reality, where not only tasks are performed but also there are unique occasions of development offered to him. The second is a spiritual reality, where time and space contain completely different living forms.

The corporeal being is the housing of the human being in his earthly life, the individuality or 'Ego' originates in the spiritual world. The human soul lives in different forms of conscience in these two worlds.

The above mentioned personalistic human image can also be characterised as follows:

A human being is neither a product of heredity (completed with possible illnesses and trauma, who can affect his corporeal being during his lifetime), nor the product of education and cultural, social influences, as pretended consecutively in nativism and empiricism (nor eventually a combination of both views), but is to be considered as a growing (evolving) being instead of a product.

The substance of mankind is precisely his personal development, driven by his 'Ego' organization. The 'Ego' organisation is characteristic of man. An animal will slavishly follow his instincts, it has to satisfy his impulses and will never wittingly put aside his emotions. On the other hand, man has the notion of self-control. Man has a self-consciousness, as proved by the fact he knows the concept 'I'. This 'Ego' organisation puts his stamp on other existential parts (namely the physical body, the mental body and the emotional body) and gradually turns every man, unto the physical-hereditary level, into an individual spiritual being.

WHAT HAPPENS FROM CONCEPTION UNTIL THE DEVELOPMENT TO A GROWN HUMAN BEING

The 'Ego', the spirit of man and also the centre of its consciousness[1] is the unique in man, that finally constructs its individual body. The occupation of a body begins at birth. It is self-evident that the unborn embryo starts living in the womb, so that human life does not begin at birth, but **at the time of birth the 'Ego' of man joins the body,** which is called incarnation.

(Hence, the importance of the correct hour and place of birth in the so-called birth-horoscope of the astrology is evident.)

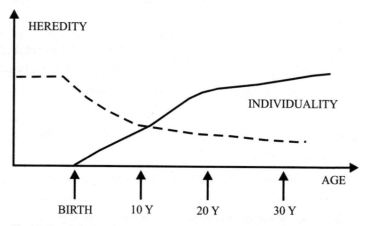

Fig. 4.1 : Transformation of the inherited substance into the individual body, (during lifetime)

After that, it takes quite some years before the new human body, born out of his mother, is drenched totally with the 'Ego' of the child because this 'I' has to transform and change the inherited

---

1. Remark: In the Jungian's view, the ego is the centre of consciousness.

substance of the body until it get built up into his own individual body[2]. Such a remodelling of matter happens as long as man lives, because untill that time he can change himself.

In such way, there are two types of powers, first which man inherits and other 'Ego' power that gradually dominates the inherited power and unfolds itself. Still these inherited powers are always present partially.

Now, the question arises, which homeopathic symptoms are correlated with the inherited factors and can be distinguished from the actual 'Ego' symptoms'?

Consequently, two remedies should come to the front, that is the individual remedy determined by the 'Ego' symptoms and the remedy related to the inherited features.

Remedies, which in homeopathy are marked by **the hereditary load are mainly the classic nosodes, being Carcinosinum, Medorrhinum, Syphilinum and Tuberculinum**.

Starting from the hypothesis, heredity reveals itself especially by the nosodal symptoms, **an artificial division of the symptoms to repertorise is made**:

1. On the one side the nosodal symptoms are placed.
2. On the other side the non-nosodal symptoms are placed. These non-nosodal symptoms consequently refer to the individual or 'Ego' symptoms.

---

2. Remark: In the Jungian's view, infants at birth are totally identified with the Self. Their sense of individuality develops later when the ego starts in his development. This is done through projection onto the parents, especially the mother, as the child grows up.

The Self is the central archetype that influences all of the archetypal energies with the purpose of moving an individual towards unity, what Jung called individuation. The Self, which encloses both conscious and unconscious, goes beyond and cannot be identified by the individual (Cicchetti, J.: Dreams, Symbols and Homeopathy).

In the hierarchy of preference to administer a homeopathic remedy, Pierre Schmidt proposed to give, if possible, first the remedy of vegetable kingdom, then of the minerals, then those of the animal kingdom and at last those coming from the mankind. The main reason is that as closer one comes to the human body, closer one comes to heredity factors (See, chapter: Classic nosodes). In this manner we can, according to what the actual condition of the patient requires, act upon the individual conditions or upon hereditary layers of the patient. This state of the patient can be examined exactly by the energetic examination, cf. Bibliography).

Mostly, if a classic nosode is indicated, it will be as an intercurrent remedy. Once the hereditary blockage is removed, one can often administer an individual remedy.

Other nosodes too, apart from the already mentioned four classic nosodes, can remove a blockage arising from family or personal antecedents, like the after-effects of vaccinations or as mentioned by Dr D. M. Foubister. Likewise, an overuse of allopathic products such as hemp, quinine, etc. can cause a blockage, which can be inherited and consequently be treated by an isopathic remedy, as mentioned by G. Vithoulkas.

The main repertorisation is thus based on the search of the simillimum that corresponds to the characteristic non-nosodal symptoms. Once the simillimum is found, we can still make a distinction of the nosodal symptoms, namely those symptoms which are also covered by the simillimum, and consequently are confirmative for the selected simillimum and the symptoms that only refer to a nosode. The predominant nosode amongst the latter group of symptoms is the most important and eventually be indicated if an intercurrent administration of the nosode during the treatment is necessary.

Sometimes, during the treatment of the patient, we find that different nosodes can be used intermediately, because most of our patients have tri-miasmatic disease.

CONCLUSION

Concerning heredity and classic nosodes (by exception of Psorinum)

1. By means of the individual simillimum we treat the totality of the patient in a correct miasmatic manner (H – § 7 and A). Masi, according to the dynamic miasmatic concept).
2. The predominance of nosodal symptoms in babies and infants is usually striking. This means that nosodes are usually more indicated in childhood as compared to adolescence. This is in accordance with the anthroposophic view.
3. Hereditary blockages can eventually be removed by the known nosodes, also by nosodes other than the classic ones.
4. In this way of repertorisation, the knowledge of the materia medica of above-mentioned nosodes is very important.

Indications for the prescription of a classic or other nosode

1. The classic indications to prescribe nosodes are based on the family and personal history, failure of related remedies though apparently well indicated, or indications for two or more of the related remedies without complete coverage by one (The Carcinosin drug picture - Dr D. M. Foubister)
2. A nosode can be indicated when the duration of action of the simillimum is too short (This is in contradiction with Kent's lecture XXXV, 5th and 6th observation).
3. From my own experience, Carcinosinum is mostly an intercurrent remedy and when given removes, immediately the hereditary layer so that the individual remedy may be administered directly after it or within a short interval (This is an exception to the rule that indicates never to give two or more deep acting remedies successively).

For example: There is a Kalium phosphoricum patient who apparently does not react on the repetition of the remedy although he always produces Kalium phosphoricum symptoms and it is really the simillimum of the patient.

Now, what to do?

Indeed at that moment it is indicated to think at the prescription of a nosode.

For example, if you think of Carcinosinum (by the family and personal history), and prescribe it, followed by a wait and watch period. Sometimes your choice is suggested and confirmed by a new symptom which contains that nosode.

Two reactions are possible:

i. Either the patient is better, then the **new symptoms** lead to the following prescription:
   a. It will be the same individual remedy as the previous one (Kalium phosphoricum).
   b. It will be another remedy:
      - A complementary remedy or a remedy that follows well
      - A remedy without any specific affinity to the previous remedy
      - A nosode (for example Psorinum)
ii. Or, the patient is not better.

NB: New symptoms again lead to the following remedy.)

Then, let's hope, Carcinosinum (if correct) had nevertheless acted and moved away the hereditary layer. When the symptoms of the patient are not changed since the intake of Carcinosinum, then Kalium phosphoricum has to be re-administered. Mostly the patient reacts well.

Illustration by using an analogous example of a wound up car

Heredity and Classic Nosodes

which gets stuck against a wall and which is restarted after the removal of the wall:

i. Car starts and moves forward.
ii. Car gets stuck against a wall and comes totally to a standstill.
iii. Removal of the wall.
iv. Car must be rewound because it came to a standstill.
v. Now, car can continue its way.

But, if there is no reaction at all, then there are also two options:

a. Either you are sure that the individual remedy is Kalium phosphoricum. Then, Psorinum can be given because it suggests that there is some hereditary blockage. If this is correct, the case will be unlocked by it's action and will now react immediately or react again after re-administering Kalium phosphorium.

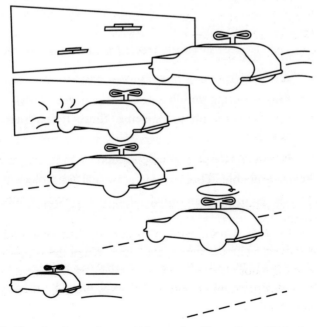

Fig. 4.2 : Illustration of a wound up car which got stuck against a wall and which has been started up again after the removal of the wall

b. Or, you have to select some other classic or bowel nosode or may be even some isopathic agent, and afterwards the case have to be reconsidered (as mentioned).

> **NB:** Or Kalium phosphoricum is not the simillimum and you have to look for another individual remedy by the guidance of some <u>new symptoms</u>.

CASES

Case 1: Girl, 6 years of age

Family anamnesis:

i. Maternal grandfather and grandmother died of cancer.
ii. Paternal grandfather died of cancer.
iii. Sister, 9 years, had Legg-Calvé-Perthes.
vi. Mother and sister successfully treated with Carcinosinum.

Personal anamnesis:

Sleeping problems during childhood. Constipation and bellyache since years, at first difficult to describe. Since a few months, daily cramping abdominal pains, especially in the evening, pain just below the navel, which was ameliorated by pressure and by slightly bending double. This attitude is typical for Colocynthis, but 'Abdomen, pain, pressure amel.' is also a nosode symptom (Carcinosinum).

During further interrogation, the patient's sister told something striking that she did not want to share the same bed with the patient anymore because the latter constantly used to kick her during sleep.

Other chronic symptoms were:

i. She loved her cat very much.
ii. She had fear in the dark.
iii. Craved icy cold milk and eggs.

Screening of the symptoms:

i. Loves animals (Carc., Med.).
ii. Fear of dark (Carc., Med.).
iii. Desires icy cold milk (Tub.).
iv. Desires eggs (Carc.).
v. Abdomen pain ameliorates by pressure (Carc.).
vi. Pain in a small spot below navel (Coloc. and Zinc from W. Boericke and Calc. from S. Hahnemann).
vii. Restlessness of lower limbs at evening and night in bed (Zincum metallicum) (Repertory of Kent).

Finally there were only two non-nosodal symptoms, which refered to Zincum metallicum. Carcinosinum was already given earlier on account of the family anamnesis, but did not cure the abdominal complaints. Taking Zincum metallicum 200 K resulted in an immediate and lasting improvement.

Nosodal symptoms, which did not contain Zincum metallicum were:

i. Loves animals.
ii. Desire for cold milk.
iii. Desire for eggs.
iv. Abdomen, pain, pressure amel.

Using these symptoms could mislead one in order to find the simillimum.

Case 2: Female 12 years of age

Family anamnesis: Negative.

Personal anamnesis:

Her mother was consulting for the patient that she was always very nervous and tense. In consequence of this, during the school year, she had sleep-walking every night, something that did not occur during the holidays. Before the examinations she used to suffer from diarrhoea. Furthermore, she was very fastidious, she used to weep at the least reprimand and she was anxious in the dark, because it felt as if there is somebody in the room. She used to avoid the sun, disliked hot drinks, loved steak and exhibited skin warts.

Screening of the symptoms:
i. Delusions, another person is in the room.
ii. Fastidious (Carc., Med.).
iii. Fear of dark (Carc., Med.).
iv. Restlessness in children (Carc., Tub.).
v. Somnambulism.
vi. Weeping, from admonitions/reprimands (Carc.).
vii. Rectum, diarrhoea from excitement (Carc.).
viii. Skin, warts (Carc., Tub.).
ix. Generalities, aversion to hot drinks.
x. Generalities, desire for meat (Tub.).
xi. Generalities, sun aggravates (Tub.).

Repertorisation of the 'non-nosodal' symptoms:
i. Delusions, another person is in the room.
ii. Somnambulism.
iii. Generalities, aversion to hot drinks.
   The remedy is Lycopodium clavatum.

Nosodal symptoms, which did not contain Lycopodium clavatum are:

i. Fastidious (Carc., Med.).
ii. Restlessness in children (Carc., Tub.).
iii. Stomach, desire for meat (Tub.).
iv. Generalities, sun aggravates (Tub.).

If we used these symptoms we could have been misled in finding the simillimum. Therefore, we have to keep in mind that every individual is suspected to be hereditary contaminated with all miasms, even when the family anamnesis is negative.

Lycopodium clavatum 200 K was administered and since then the nervousness at school and the sleep-walking completely ceased, without using a nosode.

Case 3: Woman, 42 years of age

Family anamnesis: Father died from leukaemia.

Personal anamnesis:

i. Seventh of eight children, Hepatitis B at the age of 21, contaminated while doing her medical laboratory work.
ii. Unilateral headache around the eye with nausea, mostly caused by stress, heat (for instance in a car) and especially during ovulation. Ameliorated by cold applications, darkness and eating less. On the other hand, fasting provoked the headache.
iii. Fibroma of the uterus, with diameter of 2 cm.

The patient wanted order and perfection in the household. She loves to cook and being sociable, she liked to invite people.

She liked to go to parties, to travel and prefered the sea and sun. When she was being asked something, she could hardly refuse. She was an active member in the corporate life and she liked to be held in respect.

She was very worried about her children, wanted them to be home in time (for instance to eat) and liked the house to be cosy.

She was afraid of heights (3 meter), got anxious in the car since a year.

She was a tearful baby that liked to be rocked. Timid, punctual, docile and dutiful in obeying certain rules. Sometimes she was afraid of the dark and feared that she would lose vision.

Local complaints:

i. Pain inside the ear while walking in cold wind.

Other symptoms:

i. Desired soup and dishes with vinegar. She did not like fish.
ii. Constipation before menstruation, bleeding only during daytime.
iii. Usually she used to sleep on the abdomen and preferably in pitch-darkness. She had coloured dreams, sometimes about robbers, sometimes of flying or floating.

Repertorisation of the 'non-nosodal' symptoms:

i. Menses, ceases when lying, daytime only, ceases while resting.
ii. Ovulation agg.*: Aloe, Chel., Cocc., Foll., Granit-m., Ham., Hydr., LAC-C., Lach., Mag-c., Mag-m., Meli., Merc., Nux-v., Rumx., Sacch., Sep., Sep-cal-bil., Sulph., Vanad., Vip-t.
iii. Ear pain in cold wind.
iv. Head, pain, cold applications ameliorates.
v. Mind, anxiety while riding (Lach.).
vi. Dreams, coloured (Lach.).

The repertorisation pointed to Lac caninum, taking into account its close relationship with Lachesis mutus (see, chapter: Complementary and allied remedies first edition, 1994).

Nosodal symptoms, which did not contain Lac caninum were:

i. Fastidious (Carc., Tub.).
ii. Rocking amel. (Carc.).
iii. Dreams of flying (Carc.*).
iv. Stomach, desire for soup (Carc.*).

If these symptoms were used, we could have been misled in finding the simillimum.

So, Lac caninum was prescribed and cured her without using Carcinosicum as intercurrent nosode.

Case 4: Boy, 7 years of age: Agaricus muscarius - Tuberculinum

This young boy suffered from glue ears since years, but his main complaint was a relapsing bronchitis. Every time this bronchitis was preceded by eczema and cracking of the left earlobe. When the child had fever, it was striking that his hair used to stand up in spots.

There were some remarkable aspects in his behaviour. At home he was very helpful, though he was violent while playing. On the other hand, he was very timid at school. He liked to talk big, but in fact he was weak hearted.

He desired sweet things and salty food and he was always thirsty for large quantities. He liked to be washed with cold water.

In the evening, there was sleeping with a distinct perspiration in the cervical region.

Analysis of the cases:

There were a lot of Tuberculinum symptoms, namely:

i. Ear, eruptions, crack behind ear.
ii. Stomach, thirst for large quantities.
iii. Back, perspiration of cervical region, night.
iv. Chest, inflammation, bronchial tubes.

Since the child already received several times Tuberculinum by a colleague, without apparent result, another remedy was looked out for.

Apart from that, two particular symptoms referred to Agaricus muscarius:

i. Head, stand-up spots of hair on the scalp (A. Masi).
ii. Mind, benevolence / servile*.

(Adult Agaricus muscarius patient likes to care about the sick and the dying. Agaricus children also show some of this concern and this finds expression of their helpfulness at home.)

So, the nosode took away the hereditary layer, but did not cure the patient. So, Agaricus muscarius, being complementary to Tuberculinum, was administered. Then, the tendency to bronchial inflammation, together with chronic inflammation of the ear disappeared after some doses of Agaricus muscarius.

Case 5: Man, 58 years of age: Astacus fluviatilis – Medorrhinum

Family anamnesis: Father had Dupuytren's contraction.

Personal anamnesis:

i. Recurrent colds as child.
ii. Herpes zoster at the age of 24.
iii. Cigarette smoker till the age of 37.
iv. Divorce followed by a second marriage 15 years ago.

v. Dupuytren surgery of hand.

The patient was depressive because of his work. He liked to take up a new challenge but on the other hand felt unsure. He was especially afraid of being criticized (Medorrhinum).

He was since many years a fervent amateur cyclist and affronts himself with big challenges as to ride up yearly the mount Tourmalet. Every week he cycled some hundreds of kilometres.

Now, he frequently suffered from sudden atrial tachycardia which was induced by a prolonged physical exertion as a long cycling tour. When he had that atrial tachycardia he felt some pressure in the axilla.

After sometime he was in good condition without atrial tachycardia but he consulted me for the complaint of having a plug of mucous in throat at night from which he frequently used to wake up.

By the help of energetic examination I found Astacus fluviatilis, which was administered to him in MK. A week later I saw him back very urgently. He felt really bad, had dyspnea, perspiration all over and tachycardia at the least physical exercise.

He was also mentioning of a dream he had last night. In the dream, he took pity on a homeless person and took him into his house. In the dream he was again in his parental house and he saw his father who was busy papering and painting the interior. He explored every possibility to get some job for that person, but every time he proposed him something, the man refused. Also, he did not perform anything of household affairs. This altogether made him finally so angry that he threw that person out of the door.

Chronology of the themes:

i. Theme of caring, mothering.

ii. Theme of sudden outburst of suppressed anger towards the person he took care.

Discussion:

These themes are typical of Astacus fluviatilis (cf. proving of Doris Drach and Franz Swoboda, Documenta Homoeopathica, Band 23), where a woman prover dreamt that she put her child outside of the door. Afterwards that prover was very dismayed about her own behaviour towards her child in the dream because she surely would never do such a thing because normally she had strong concern for her children and had very strong motherly feelings.

As a reaction on the correct administration of Astacus fluviatilis, probably an ancestral hereditary blockage was risen.

Because the complaints were especially centred around the heart Medorrhinum was the first nosode to think of. Also, his sensitivity to criticism led into that direction. Also, the energetic examination confirmed that hypothesis and consequently Medorrhinum, XMK was administered to the patient.

Reaction and follow-up:

The same day of administration of the remedy the tachycardia stopped and the patient again acquired the good condition. Since that day he never had attacks of tachycardia and also the lump sensation at night was gone.

Case 6: Boy, 14 years of age: Cisplatina - Tuberculinum

(See chapter: Classic nosodes: Common features of the ancestral energy out of balance).

Chapter 5

Nosodes

DEFINITION

Nosodes are the remedies which are made of bacteria and viruses, diseased tissue, excretions or mixtures of these. Some of them have been proved and others have not. They are supposed to contain the signature of the disease.

HISTORY

Hahnemann did not know the concept of 'nosode' but he had an acquaintance with isopathic agents. He did a proving of the sero-purulent matter of a scabies vesicle, 'wet psora'. This experiment was published by Stapf in 1833. Then, the first nosode 'Psorinum' was know.

The product 'dry psora' taken from the epidermoid efflorescence of pityriasis was used by Gross to make another proving of Psorinum.

In the year 1833, Hering introduced the nosode 'Lyssinum'. In 1854, a Brazilian homeopath had the first proving with the sputum of T.B. patient, which led to the full proving of Tuberculinum. In 1880, Swan published the provings of Medorrhinum and Syphilinum. Shortly after, Burnett published the proving of

Bacillinum in 1885. Kent introduced the nosode Carcinosinum. The Bowel nosodes were introduced by Edward Bach in 1920. Deeper research about Carcinosinum was done by Foubister and Templeton in 1952.

INDICATIONS TO PRESCRIBE A NOSODE

1. The classic indications to prescribe nosodes are mainly based on the family and personal anamnesis:
    i. The family anamnesis especially indicates to classic nosodes (cf. page 54 Indications for the prescription of a classic or other nosode).
    ii. The personal anamnesis indicates more towards isopathic nosodes (cf. page 55 Medorrhinum, case 2, comment).
2. Nosodes are indicated in chronic cases when well selected remedies fail to relieve or permanently cure (cf. Allen, H.C., The Materia Medica of the Nosodes, in the introduction of Psorinum).
3. A classic nosode can be prescribed as the 'fundamental' homeopathic remedy of a patient on the basis of its indications. This possibility is very rare.
4. A nosode, especially Psorinum, can be used to finish a constitutional treatment. This is the way I mostly use classic nosodes.
5. A nosode can also be used:
    i. To clarify an unclear remedy picture: This is the indication to prescribe a Bowel nosode.
    ii. To remove a blockage: This is the indication to prescribe an isopathic agent. Sometimes there is also a notion of 'Never well since'.
    iii. As a prophylactic remedy, for example during a severe flu epidemic.

Chapter 6

Classic Nosodes

The classic nosodes, as I already had mentioned, have a specific **relation with heredity**. It means that their energy acts especially upon some extra-channels (vessels or meridians), which transport inheritable forces, the ancestral energy. These forces are bounded with the chromosomes and they come from our ancestors. So, it is not something particular of the individual but common to a large number of his relatives (cf. epigenetic: see chapter: Heredity, introduction). This explains why the **family anamnesis** is so important for selecting a nosode.

Pierre Schmidt proposed a hierarchy to administer in preference of our homeopathic remedies. Namely, first the remedy of vegetable kingdom, then of the minerals, then those of the animal kingdom and at last those coming from the mankind. To understand this, one can say that as closer one comes to the human being, more closer one comes to the identical and consequently to the similar.

The ancestral energy determines a great part our immune system and life force and explains the tendencies to illnesses in the form of so-called congenital weakness. This energy is especially transported by the Conception and Governing Vessel.

So, we can prove that each one of the classic nosodes, **by exception of Psorinum**, has a disturbance of this energy system.

This can be verified by the energetic examination by making use of muscle-tests.

Every muscle of our body gets an energy from a specific acupuncture meridian. Thus, a specific meridian-function can be tested indirectly by its related muscle.

All of them, by exception of Psorinum, have a **TL on Conception Vessel 24**, which is especially related to the hereditary ancestral energy of the Conception Vessel. Psorinum also has a disturbance of the ancestral energy, but in another way (see chapter: Psora and nosodes).

Abbreviations of the different Carcinosinums:

- CARC.: All carcinosinums
- Carc.: Carcinosinum of Kent (from the United States of an unknown origin, probably prepared from an epithelioma of the breast)
- Carc-bl-adp.: Carcinosinum bladder adeno papillar
- Carc-col-ad.: Carcinosinum colon adeno
- Carc-col-adp.: Carcinosinum colon adeno papillar
- Carc-f.: Carcinosinum foubister
- Carc-in.: Carcinosinum intestines co
- Carc-lu-ads.: Carcinosinum lung adeno squamous
- Carc-mamm.: Carcinosin mammae
- Carc-rec-ad.: Carcinosinum rectum adeno
- Carc-st-ad.: Carcinosinum stomach adeno
- Carc-st-sc.: Carcinosinum stomach scirrhus
- Carc-ut-ad.: Carcinosinum uterus adeno
- Scir.: Scirrhinum (the nosode of the scirrhous cancer of the liver)
- ( ) : Bilaterally possible, yet only at one side in the patient

Classic Nosodes 93

- E.C.: Patient with eyes closed
- E.O.: Patient with eyes open
1. **Supraspinatus** (relation with the Conception Vessel):
    i. LEFT : E.O. : (Med.), Tub-m., V-a-b.
        a. Little finger upward:
            E.C. : (Carc-bl-adp.), (Med.), Syph., Tub-d., Tub-m.
        b. Thumb upward:
            E.C.: Carc-st-ad.,(Carc-f.), V-a-b.
    ii. RIGHT : E.O.: Bac., CARC., (Med.), Scir., Tub-a., Tub., Tub-burnett, Tub-d., Tub-k. Tub-r., Tub-sp.
        E.C. : Carc-in., V-a-b.
        a. Little finger upward:
            E.C.: (Carc-f.), (Carc-bl-adp.), (Med.), Tub-a., Tub-k., Tub-r.
        b. Thumb upward:
            E.O.: Syph.
            E.C.: Carc., (Carc-f.), Tub.
2. **Teres major** (relation with the Governing Vessel):
    i. LEFT : E.C.: Carc., Carc-st-ad., Tub-a.
    ii. RIGHT : E.C.: Bac., Tub-r., Carc-bl-adp.
    iii. Bilaterally, simultaneous: Syph. (E.C.).
3. Carcinosinum acts on the KIDNEY-energy:
    i. CARC.: Right m. psoas (E.C.).
    ii. Carc-lu-ads.: Left m. trapezius, upper portion (E.O.).
4. Medorrhinum acts on the Heart-energy:
    i. Right m. subscapularis (E.C.).
5. Syphilinum acts on the LIVER-energy:
    i. Left or right m. rhomboideus (E.C.).
    ii. Left or right m. pectoralis major - pars sternalis (E.C.).

6. <u>Tuberculinum</u> acts on the LUNG-energy:
   i. Bac.: Right m. coracobrachialis (E.C.).
   ii. Tub.: Left m. deltoideus medius (E.C).
       Right m. coracobrachialis (E.O.).
   iii. Tub-a.: Left m. deltoideus medius (E.C.)
   iv. Tub-burnett: Left m. deltoideus medius (E.O.)
   v. Tub-d.: Right m. serratus anterior (E.O.).
       Left m. deltoideus medius (E.O.).
   vi. Tub-k.: Left or right m. deltoideus medius (E.C.).
       Left or right m. serratus anterior (E.C.).
   vii. Tub-m.: Left or right m. deltoideus medius (E.C.).
       Left or right m. deltoideus posterior (E.O.).
       Right m. brachioradialis (E.O.).
   viii. Tub-r.: Hypertonic left m. tensor fasciae latae (E.C.).
   ix. Tub-sp. : Left or right m. serratus anterior (E.C.).
       Left or right m. coracobrachialis (E.C.).

Other weakened muscles and energetic points:
1. Carcinoisum:
   i. Left m. deltoideus anterior (E.O.).
   ii. Left m. rhomboideus (E.O.), except carc-col-ad.
   iii. Carc-col-ad. : Left m. gluteus maximus.
   iv. Carc-lu-ads.: Left m. trapezius, upper portion (E.C.).
   v. Scir. : Left m. coracobrachialis (E.C.).
       Left m. soleus (E.C.).
       Right m. trapezius, lower portion (E.C.).
2. Medorrhinum:
   i. Left m. latissimus dorsi (E.O.).
   ii. Left or right m. infraspinatus (E.C.).
   iii. Left or right m. rhomboideus (E.C.).

3. Syphilinum:
   i. Right m. latissimus dorsi (E.O.).
4. Tuberculinum:
   i. Tub-burnett: Left m. gluteus medius (E.O.).
   ii. Tub.m.: Left or right m. teres minor (E.C.).
       Right m. brachioradialis (E.O.).
   iii. V-a-b. : Right m. rhomboideus (E.O.).
        Left m. gluteus maximus (E.O.).
        Mm. recti abdomini, lower part, bilaterally (E.O.).

SCREENING OF THE CLASSIC NOSODES BY ENERGETIC POINTS

Carcinosinum

1. Weihe Point:

    Carcinosinum itself has no W.P. However, it changes the laterality of the magnetic field of the body. When we examine the W.P. of the associated constitutional remedy, we find it on the hetero-lateral side. Also its physiognomy get changed from laterality.

    For example, when Lycopodium clavatum is the associated constitutional remedy, we find the W.P. on the 'left' second intercostal space and the hypertonic muscule trapezius - pars descendens, situated now on the 'left' side.

2. Therapy Localization :

    There is a special handmode for Carcinosinum (see Fig. 6.1). The Carcinosinum point is situated on the convex line in the middle between the right ear and the caudal extension of the sutura sagittalis under the linea nuchae suprema.

    When holding this point with the middle and index fingertip in superposition, the indicator muscle becomes weak.

    Another point is situated on the left third rib, on the parasternal line*.

    Sometimes, with constitutional screening find a combination of Calcarea phosphoria and Calcarea carbonica*.

    Sometimes when holding the hand with the emotional handmode (with spread fingers) on the umbilicus, the strong indicator muscle becomes weak. Sometimes the TL on the 'cancer-points, Bladder 12 and 38' are positive, bilaterally.

Carc-rec-ad.: Switching of cerebral hemispheres in a sequence of 3/1;3/1;3/1; etc. Energetic point: N-UE-26, on the right side.

Carc-st-sc.: Energetic points on the left side: N-BW-23 (left) and Lung 2. Sensitivity of the third cervical nerve, on the right side.

Scirrhinum: Energetic points on N-UE-26 and on the right side Bladder 56, bilaterally.

Medorrhinum

1. Weihe Point:
   The W.P. of Medorrhinum is situated in the middle of the left calf (Bladder 58).
2. Therapy Localization :
   There is a special handmode for Medorrhinum (Bladder 58, bilaterally). See Fig. 6.2.

> **NB:** The same handmode is seen in case of Morgan Pure (Paterson) (see chapter: Bowel nosodes.)

Another Medorrhinum point is situated behind the right processus mastoideus (cf. Thuja occidentalis).

Syphilinum

1. Weihe Point :
   Bladder 39 can be used (bilaterally). This point is situated at the middle of the hollow of knee.
2. Therapy Localization :
   There is a special handmode for Syphilinum (see fig.6.3).

> **NB :** The same handmode is seen in case of Gaertner (Bach) (see chapter: Bowel nosodes.)

The Syphilinum point is situated on the back of the left processus mastoideus (cf. Mercurius solubilis).

Sometimes, by constitutional screening, we find the same as found in Calcarea fluorica*.

Tuberculinum

1. Weihe Point:

   The point on the anterior surface of the sternum between the W.P.'s of Argentum metallicum and Phosphorus can be used as W.P.

2. Therapy Localization :

   There is a special handmode for Tuberculinum (see fig. 6.4).

> **NB :** The same handmode is seen in case of Bacillus 7 (Paterson) (see chapter: Bowel nosodes).

The Tuberculicum point is situated on two inch distance from the anterior fontanelle, on the left side, laterally except for Tub-r. which point is situated at the right side.

Tuberculinum marmoreck : Right Bladder 23 and Bladder 44, bilaterally.

Tub-sp.: Right N-UE-26 (E.O.) and right Liver 2 (E.C.).

V-a-b.: Left N-BW 14 (E.O.).

Classic Nosodes

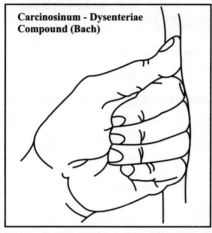

Fig. 6.1: Handmode of Carcinosinum (MD: T2, 3 and IMRL 7, 8 to skin, -IMRL)

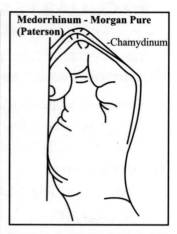

Fig. 6.2: Handmode of Medorrhinum (MD: IMRL/T against skin)

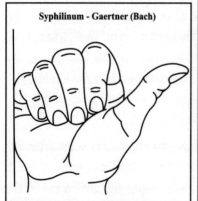

Fig. 6.3: Handmode of Syphilinum (MD: -IMRL, OT, lateral aspect of hand to skin)

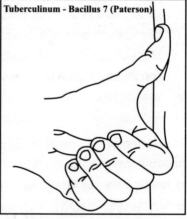

Fig. 6.4: Handmode of Tuberculinum (MD: T2T3Ib-skin, -IMRL)

PECULIAR FEATURES OF CLASSIC NOSODES

Common Features

1. Despair of recovery (Psorinum), even the patient says that he is very sick when he is going better (Carcinosinum, Medorrhinum, Syphilinum). Tuberculinum has no despair of recovery.
2. Underlying feeling: If life ends, there is nothing after.
3. Want of identity.

   The nosode of a miasm, for example, Psorinum (Psora), Medorrhinum (Sycosis) or Syphilinum (Syphilis) represents the centre-point of a miasm. The nosode is the disease product which is made from the tissue that is fully under the influence of the infection. **This tissue is so completely overcome by the infection that it is no longer in it the individuality of the person**, but only under the signs of the process of the infection. (Sankaran, R., The Substance of Homoeopathy)

4. Fixed ideas, persistent thoughts.

   The nosode of a miasm, for example, Psorinum (Psora), Medorrhinum (Sycosis) or Syphilinum (Syphilis) represents the centre-point of a miasm. The nosode is the disease product which is made from the tissue that is fully under the influence of the infection. This tissue is so completely overcome by the infection that it is no longer in it the individuality of the person, but only under the signs of the process of the infection. (Sankaran, R., The Substance of Homoeopathy)

Carcinosinums

Carcinosinum (Kent)

- **A Carcinosinum patient cannot differentiate himself because he is too tightly connected with his family**
- **Secretive people** who have problems to communicate their inner feelings about some bad experiences in their youth, because they have the feeling that they cannot tell everything about their family. They are cooped in themselves and feel themselves martyrs
- **Over-responsible yet romantic people**
- **Needs having 'control' over everything what happens**
- **The nucleus idea of Carcinosinum is that he has the feeling that he himself has not chosen his life. So, he has to undergo life or he has to rebel.**

  In Carcinosinum there is tendency to crucifixion and self-effacing (Carcinosin cannot say 'no'). They fail to adapt themselves to new situations and evolutions. They hold too strong to old-fashioned values (impressed by their education). See also in the chapter of miasms and their psychological background.

  Helmut Ossege compares Carcinosinum people with angels.

  Angels have no personal longings and needs. They come to us to help and sacrify themselves

- **Reverence for nature forces and technology**: Carcinosinum patient gets goose flesh when he sees an athlete breaking a record, an impressive waterfall or a take-off of an airplane
- The typical Carcinosinum appearance is: Blue sclerotics, a brownish café-au-lait complexion, moles, naevi, bizarre tics, grimaces, blinking of the eyes, scraping the throat before being able to speak, etc

- Injury of head during parturition
- Sleeplessness with weeping in newborns
- Child must be rocked
- Deep-seated throbbing headache
- Injury of the head, e.g. during birth
- Growth of hair on tongue. Absence of papillae at tip of tongue
- Acidosis
- Pain in region above the umbilicus
- Symphysiolysis (during pregnancy)
- Asthma from fright
- Every heartbeat is felt in the whole body
- Pain at cervical region on the right side, which aggravates when turning the head to the right
- Dream: Looking for someone and failing to find that person e.g. a partner to marry with however the dreamer is already married
- Amelioration during the evening
- Waking at 4 a.m.
- **Amelioration in tiredness from physical exertion, e.g. jogging**
- Auto-immune diseases
- Never well since mononucleosis
- Chronic fatigue syndrome
- Autism*
- Food: Eating in succession each kind of food apart
- Warm-blooded

The new preparations of Carcinosinum (Foubister)

Carc-bl-adp., Carc-col-ad., Carc-col-adp., Carc-f., Carc-in., Carc-lu-ads., Carc-mamm., Carc-rec-ad., Carc-st-ad., Carc-st-sc., Carc-ut-ad. The new preparations are very potent and can cause violent reactions.

Indications to prescribe them:

There must be a specific location of some complaints in the personal or family history. Example: from the British Homoeopathic Journal, vol. XLVII, July 1958, no. 3, The Carcinosin Drug Picture, D.M. Foubister, there is a case where Carc-st-ad. is selected because of fright in the stomach and vomiting on anticipation.

Or, there is a peculiar symptom which refers to that specific Carcinosinum. Example: Carc-rec-ad. dreams of a sunken or low (interior) wall which reach only half the height of a normal one*.

Scirrhinum (Burnett)

The picture of Scirrhinum closely resembles **Phosphorus**:

- Thin built and **chilly**
- Strong desire for cold drinks
- Many fears
- Keynote symptom: Sinking sensation at the navel (Kalium carbonicum, Phosphorus)

Other strong symptoms are:

- Haemorrhoids and sometimes a chronic, necrotic haemorrhoidal mass
- Haemorrhages and varicosis of legs and feet with purple discolouration
- Glandular affections
- Cancer of breast
- Stony hard glands and lumps
- Threadworms (in children), they crawl out at 5-6 p.m. and not during the night
- Aggravation from 5 to 6 p.m.

Medorrhinum
- Medorrhinum patients are hurried and are continuously occupied with what they have to do in the near future. They are self-centred
- Anticipation
- **Bulldozer-type children**
- People with an extreme behaviour at all levels
- Inflammation of ring holes of ears
- Perspiration on face and upper lip
- Biting tip of tongue during sleep
- Can only pass stool by leaning far backward
- Chronic pelvic disorders of women
- **Endometriosis**
- **Lumbago and sciatica resemble a Rhus toxicodendron picture**
- Hairy arms
- Medorrhinum patients frequently scrape the throat (Carcinosinum)
- Asthma at 2 a.m.
- Itching without eruptions
- **Heart** complaints
- Pain in heart from apex to base (Syphilinum has the reverse)
- Pain in kidney region which ameliorates after urination
- **Lumbago and sciatica, resembling a Rhus toxicodendron picture** (Pladys Albert)
- Sensitiveness of soles or feet

Psorinum
- Psorinum people are born losers who are helplessly under the sway of the ups and downs of life (Vermeulen Frans)

- Introverted and pessimistic people who feels themselves separated and have an unreasonable fright and fear of everything
- Fear of poverty, failure, health and future
- People who are fixed at the oral stage of Freud's psychosexual development (Grandgeorge Didier)
- People having an inferiority complex
- Unhealthy looking children. Early senescence in children
- Greasy face, especially greasy perspiration on the forehead. Hair growth on the face
- Allergy
- Hay fever
- Very chilly people having an intolerance of woollen clothes
- Amelioration while lying on the back during:
  - Heart pain
  - Cough and asthma ameliorates when lying on back with arms spread out 'as if crucified'

Syphilinum

- Observation: Parallel lines never touch each other (Sherr Jeremy)
  - Linear headache, commencing at both angles of forehead and extending in parallel lines backward
  - Red and indented tongue with two deep cracks running lengthwise on each side of median line
- Keynote (by extrapolation): Symbolic **wish of 'meeting each other'**(Sherr Jeremy), which never happens and consequently creates mental despair (cf. washing always the hands)
- Delusion of being dirty and fear of becoming contaminated so that one washes always the hands

- Pathology at meeting points:
  - Inner canthi of eyes
  - Dwarfed teeth converge at their tips
  - Pain in heart from base to apex (Medorrhinum has the reverse)
- Headache from temple to temple, deep into brain from vertex or region above the eye
- Hair becomes prematurely gray (Sycotic co.)
- Calcareous deposits on tympanum
- Children's teeth are cupped
- Sensitiveness of os uteri e.g. during p.p.v. or coition
- Perspiration between scapulae
- **Crying babies from birth**, lasting for months and even till the age of 2
- Night aggravation

Tuberculinum

The common picture of Tuberculinum fits best with the picture of Tuberculinum bovinum Koch because its materia medica is the most extensive of all the Tuberculinums, yet all the symptoms of all Tuberculinums must be considered to create the whole picture.

- Keynotes: Tuberculinum people live **like a candle which burns at both ends** (Vithoulkas, George) because they have the sensation that life is very short and they have to live very intensely
- Tuberculinum is indicated in a case which needs to be oxigenized, that means the patient is weak and needs more air, oxygen and freedom

Differences and discussion of each of the Tuberculinum nosodes

The following indications are not totally specific for each of them. They show the core of the action field of each of them. On condition that some other symptoms of the patient belong to the common picture of Tuberculinum, the more specific Tuberculinum can be prescribed.

Bacillinum (Burnett)
- Family history (Master Farokh):
  - Abusive parents, neglect from parents
  - Struggling parents in their own professional life and hence unable to devote enough time to their child
- Personal history:
  - Suited to 'excited' and 'restless' people
  - **Snappish**, irritability and crankiness better by being carried
  - Spitting
  - **Indifference to people around including family members (Syphilinum)**
  - **Refuses to take medicine**
  - Thoughts about constriction and about being constricted. Relating too closely to oneself without reference to anything bigger, living in a microcosm
- Especially indicated when one has to create an elimination outwards, e.g. when a lung problem (a cyst) begins after administration of Tuberculinum, Bacillinum can resolve it and brings out an elimination, eczema or diarrhoea
- Clinical observations:
  - Boils at nostrils (Hirudo medicinalis)
  - **Blepharitis**

- Eczema of margins of eyelids
- Vomiting is impossible (Belladonna, Lac defloratum)
- Pain in rectum on sneezing (Lachesis mutus)
- Accelerated respiration which ameliorates when spoken to (Master Farokh)
- Violent spasmodic cough with jerking of head forward and knees upward
- Chronic pulmonary non-tubercular diseases: Bronchial catarrh with scanty expectoration of **equally poly-bacillary elements**, chest-catarrh in old people, **humid asthma**
- Cough is from the right lung, feels like asthma with a **sensation of constriction and strangulation** with pain. At the beginning of the cough there is a significant pain at the seventh dorsal vertebra
- Dorsal vertebrae are wet and feel cold
- Pain in knees ameliorated by continued motion
- Sleep: Continuation of the former dream on going to sleep
- Bony eminences and long bones are painful to touch
- **Hot patient wants fan or air-conditioner constantly even during fever** (Master Farokh)
- Desire for vinegar which he even drinks from the bottle. Aversion to chicken

Tuberculinum bovinum (Kent)

- Keynote: Acts primarily on **the immune system** and secondly on the hormonal system
- Suited to plethoric people, who are tired and very susceptible to take cold
- Cases with:
    - Auto-immune diseases, i.e. Crohn's disease, rheumatism, etc. (Lanthanides)

- Allergy (especially to cow's milk and cats' hair), asthma, hay fever, nasal problems, rash and eczema
- Clinical observations:
  - Perforation in membrana tympani with ragged edges
  - Periodic headache with pain in neck (Silicea terra)
  - Perspiration on nose
  - Inguinal glands
  - Chronic diarrhoea in children
  - Constipation
  - **Oxyuris**
  - Tuberculous peritonitis with ascites or adhesions
  - Relaxed scrotum
  - Dysmenorrhoea: Too frequent and copious menses

Tuberculinum koch

- Keynote: Acts primarily on the **thyroid gland**
- Suited to weakened and lean person with small chest, who need to move (cf. state of hyperthyroidism)
- Clinical observations:
  - Headache of students
  - Difficult dentition
  - Pale lips with **vertical cracks**
  - Appetite increased with emaciation
  - **Diarrhoea**
  - Chronic appendicitis
  - Inguinal glands
  - Acute and chronic parenchymatous nephritis
  - Asthma
  - Broncho-pneumonia and **lobular-pneumonia**
  - Chronic rheumatism with ankylosis

- **Dry** eruptions, eczema and **fungoid** infections

Tuberculium denys
- Keynote: Acts primarily on **the hormonal system** and also on the mucous membranes
- Suited to **hydrogenoid plethoric people**, who look healthy but are little fat (obese), because they eat too much
- Clinical observations:
  - Constipation
  - Asthma
  - Phthisis pulmonalis **florida**
  - Swelling of mammae before menses
  - Arthritis deformans
  - Chronic effects of influenza poisoning
  - Recurrent colds
  - **Sudden and violent fits**, migraine, coryza, gastritis, diarrhoea, asthma, eczema, weakness, etc. E.g.: sudden weakness in (pre) tuberculous persons, who are subjected to digestive troubles, as of weakening diarrhoea, anorexia and hypotension

Tuberculinum marmoreck
- Suited to tired and lean persons with little appetite
- They are worse from exercise and better when resting
- Especially indicated in (pre)tuberculous affections and in incipient phthisis pulmonalis in young people
- There is emaciation, anorexia, adenopathy, a reversion of the Mantoux test, constipation without reason, hazy tips of lungs (on X-ray), etc.
- Personal history: Antecedents of otitis media
- Clinical observations:

- Acute otitis media in emaciated children
- Small and dry lips
- **Constipation**
- **Asthma** alternating with **wandering rheumatism**
- **Dry skin**

Tuberculinum Spengler

- Especially suited to:
  - **Pregnant women** or chlorotic **young girls**, who have weakness and fever before menses
  - **Obese** women (Calcarea carbonica)
- Clinical observations:
  - Anaemia
  - Anaemia in tuberculous patients
  - Biting lower lip while eating

Tuberculinum Avis

- Keynote: Acts primarily on the left **ear** and also on apices of lungs and kidneys
- Indicated in acute states, especially with **pulmonary congestion** and in chronic states like asthma in children
- Indicated in influenzal bronchitis
- Family history (Master Farokh):
  - There is lack of support from the father's side towards responsibilities that goes in upbringing of the child
  - There is usually a suppressed mother by dominating husband or farther-in-law or mother-in-law
  - Hyperanxious mother who is over burdened with responsibilities
- Personal history (Master Farokh):
  - Ailments from domination to the mother during pregnancy

- **Desired to be carried constantly**
- Clinical observations:
  - Acute otitis media
  - Acute broncho-pulmonary diseases of children
  - Acute inflammatory incessant cough
  - Cough after measles
  - Influenzal bronchitis
  - Weakness with anorexia

Tuberculinum residuum (Koch)

- Keynote: Acts primarily on the fibrous tissues and produces fibro-chondro-osteo-mesenchymatic **sclerosis**
- Lean and weak people with **grey** colour of face and blue lips
- Clinical observations:
  - Cracks on external third of upper lip. Dry cracked lower lip
  - Vision, dim, winking eyes ameliorates
  - Bleeding gums
  - Cicatrices
  - Congestion of veins of lower limbs
  - **Dupuytren's contraction**
  - **Chronic rheumatism** with ankylosis
  - **Acne tuberosa on back and shoulders**
  - Dry and unhealthy skin
  - **Anergy**
- Amelioration from rest and **stretching**. Evening and night amelioration
- Craving coffee
- Thirstless during fever, desire for uncovering and wants to be fanned yet the surface is cold

V-A-B. (Vaccin atténué bilié)

- Especially indicated when there is a general reaction after BCG vaccination, or after diagnostic application of the Mantoux test or Cuti-test
    - BCG vaccination: The BCG vaccine (Bacillus Calmette-Guerin) is a live, attenuated strain of bovine tubercle bacilli and has been widely used in many countries to induce specific immunity against tuberculosis. Cuti or scratch test (von Pirquet): Three scratches of 1 cm are made on the arm and one drop of crude tuberculin is put in contact with the upper and lowest scratch
    - Mantoux test: Intradermal injection of 1/10 ml PPD (purified protein derivate of tuberculin)
- Clinical observations:
    - Exaggerating symptoms
    - Excitement while reading, especially in a foreign language
    - Forgetfulness of words while speaking
    - Fear of death, of impending death
    - Delusion as if he is about to die
    - **Cracks at perineum:** Longitudinal cracks along raphe, cracks **at labia**
    - Stretching ameliorates

COMMON FEATURES OF ANCESTRAL ENERGY OUT OF BALANCE

When we look at the ancestral energy via the related classic nosodes like Psorinum, Medorrhinum, Syphilinum, Carcinosinum and Tuberculinum which express the core of each miasm, we come to the following themes by group analysis:

1. **Ego weakness (cf. Graphites)**: Ancestral blockages interfere with the development of the self-conscious, want of individuality. (cf. Degroote, F.: Notes on Miasms and Heredity (1994): All ancestral meridians, with exception of the Governing and the Conception Vessel, do not have an individual course but they use the points which belong to other meridians).
2. **Work**: Being industrious is an escape from the reality (hinc et nunc) and from own emotions and problems.
3. **Power**: An excess or a lack.
4. **Sex - sexuality - procreation**.
5. **Supernatural** forces, magic.
6. **Illness**: People who need a nosode tend to identify themselves too much with their illness, as if their own personality does not exist anymore. Stress and anticipation cause these illnesses and because of which they do not live in the reality (hinc et nunc).
7. Travelling: It is also an escape from the reality (hinc et nunc) and oneself.

Because of the ego weakness these people often <u>act as a sounding board</u> for their circle of relatives and acquaintances. So, they easily take over their regulations.

That is why we often find nosodes in defective cases where characteristic feature is a lack of peculiar and individual symptoms. By giving the appropriate nosode it happens frequently that such cases unblock and open for deeper treatment.

Psoric miasm

Discussion as per theme of the psoric miasm in context with dreams of Psorinum:

> **NB:** The real themes of Psorinum can be only detected in cases where Psorinum is prescribed as a 'single' individual remedy.

1. **Theme 1: Poverty, coldness,** being **expelled** from the Garden of Eden (Psora is the breach between man and God).

   Case 1:
   A 37-year-old woman had gastrointestinal complaints after consumption of coffee and chocolate and also in the evening after dinner. Shortly after each meal she had frequent eructations and felt very languid.

   She had dreamt about that she lived in a rented house. Outside the sun is shining, but the automatic roll-down shutters do not work. The system is blocked and the roll-down shutters are closed so that she stays 'dark' inside the house. (1)

   In another dream she lived once again in a rented house. The owner tells her that he wants to place an ornament on the wall just next to the stairs. It does not bother her as long as he does it himself. (2)

   Symptoms:
   i. Mind, delusion of being doomed and separated (1).
   ii. Mind, delusion of being poor (2).
   The key of Psorinum is poverty inside and outside.

   (cf: Kent, Lectures: For Psorinum there is no sun behind the clouds; Materia Medica, T.F. Allen: 'Sensation when the sun shines upon her as if it pushed her down, she has to rest in the shade in order to walk on.')
   Prescription: Psorinum XMMK.

   Case 2:
   A 15-year-old girl dreamt that her mother had hit a woman

with her car. Because this woman was suffering from her back, they had to pay her all the incurred medical expenses regarding her illness. Since then they could not afford any luxury at home anymore.

Prescription: Psorinum LMMK.

Case 3:

Another 40-year-old patient had a thyroid cyst accompanied with an increased thyroid activity.

She dreamt that she lived in a very big comfortless house. She felt lost in it (Comment: This big comfortless house refers to 'the chilliness and the absence of warmth' all around her. It suggests both physical and relational chilliness).

Prescription: Psorinum 6 LM, daily for one month.

Follow-up: One month after the intake of this remedy, she was now a lot more quiet and the thyroid tests were all normal.

2. **Theme 2: Impurity**

The word 'psora' was used for the first time in the Old Testament and referred to a skin disease and to the breach between God and man. Psora in that context was a punishment from God, whereby man became unclean.

The patient of case 1 had also the following dream: She dreamt that a control team of the government (in this case synonymous with God) visits to check the hygienic state inside her house. They take several samples for analysis. If the degree of dirtiness reaches a certain limit, they have to come back again. On the moment of the inspection there are visitors in the house. Promptly they hide a few chickens. However, she knows that her house is not clean enough and that the team probably would come back.

Symptoms:

i. Delusion, her house is impure.
ii. Delusion she is doomed.

Symbolically, your house in a dream is the symbol of your own body. Moreover it is said that the body is weak and impure. This reasoning is present in the extrapolation of our Christian background and stigmatizes the body as bestial and impure.

3. **Theme 3**: Being **doomed**, having no future and no hope.

   Case 4:

   A 42-year-old man dreamt about a point of assembly (stable) to deport children to concentration camps. From time to time, he takes the chance to help a child going into hiding when some conditions occur, e.g. when a child stands somewhat apart. In the dream there is never a group of children visible. On a certain moment he finds himself in a fenced-off area with high heaps of earth everywhere. He has to find his way out by following narrow paths.

   Comment:

   'Having now and then the opportunity to save someone from one's doom' refers to Psorinum because Psorinum finds oneself in a desperate situation, without any hope.

   Prescription: Psorinum MK.

   Case 5:

   A woman dreamt that an evacuation is taking place in army trucks and in that place a lot of people are gathered together. Her aunt (who died about five months ago) is sitting next to the truck driver which is now leaving. Her aunt passes her an orange wrapped in a paper through the window. When she opens the paper, she sees an orange fruit with white rotten spots.

   Comment:

   The only thing one has and which can be given is a piece of rotten fruit. This refers to Psorinum because of the aspect which is associated with poverty and impurity.

On the other hand the rotten orange refers also to the bible story about the Fall of Adam and Eve in which by the acceptance of the apple from the snake man has turned oneself away from God.

Case 6:

A 29-year-old woman dreamt that she is admitted to a hospital. She notices that the mattress of her bed, which is covered with a sheet, is soiled with dried stool. She draws the nurses attention to that fact but they act as if they do not see it. Though she is worried and a little bit upset, they ignore her.

Symptoms:

i. Mind, forsaken feeling.
ii. Dreams, stool.

Also the patient of case 3 has an analogical dream. She dreamt that she goes to the toilet to defaecate. Once in the toilet, defaecation keeps going, even in such a way that the toilet almost overflows.

Comment:

Stool refers in popular superstition to 'money', or in case of Psorinum to the shortage of money (poverty).

Symbolically defecation refers to liberation of guilt. For Psorinum this can metaphysically be related to the original sin.

A Psorinum patient has in reality often a distended abdomen, called in the German language 'der Kotbauch' (according to the diagnostic of F.X. Mayr). The belly is distended because of remaining food in the intestinal tract. Psorinum feels better, just like Calcarea carbonica, Carbo vegetabilis and Mercurius solubilis, during the constipation. In this dream we see on the contrary a drastic reversal of the typical 'reflex to retain everything' of Psorinum.

4. **Theme 4: Failure and despair.**
   Case 7:
   A 48-year-old teacher, who suffered a few months ago from lumbar pain and to whom I prescribed 'Sulphur', was visiting me because of an annoying watery coryza. This dripping of nose was lasting already for two weeks during the day and only stopped when he lay down.
   Also he told some remarkable dreams:
   i.   He constantly dreamt that he has to be present somewhere at an arranged time. When he was on the way and approaches the agreed place, he does not succeed to find the exact street however he goes there often. Finally he becomes desperate by seeking again and again without success.
   ii. In another dream he is sitting in the middle of the road trying to push himself forward. But because he gets stuck with his boots in a groove filled with mud he cannot progress due to the fact that he has to push the whole content of the groove.
   iii. In another dream he is in a Christian burial of his mother (who died some years ago). Something striking is that no one else is present in the church. Then, all of a sudden, he realizes that he neglected or forgot a lot of things during the preparation of the funeral.
   Symptoms:
   i.   Mind, anxiety of conscience.
   ii. Mind, despair.
   iii. Mind, fear of failure in business.
   iv. Mind, forsaken feeling.
   v.   Mind, mistakes in localities.
   vi. Nose, coryza, lying ameliorates (Merc., Psor.).
   vii. Dreams, unsuccessful efforts.
   Prescription: Psorinum XMMK.

Sycotic miasm

The sycotic miasm is usually compared with a blown up frog. Towards the environment one tries to give a firm impression, but in reality one is only a blown up soap bubble. That's why inside there is the feeling of being empty and fragile, which refers to an Ego weakness. This weakness is also reflected in the present anticipation, fear of being criticized and fear of an impending disease.

This results in a compensatory behaviour of being industrious and travelling (cf. Sankaran: 'I am OK as long as my weakness is covered up').

llustration by cases of Medorrhium which reflects the core of the sycotic miasm:

1. **Theme: Exaggeration**

Case 1:

A 47-year-old single woman suffered from redness about the anus. Some months ago she reacted very well on Apis mellifica.

Meanwhile she had the following dreams:

i. She has to go to the toilet and she finds the toilet is painted blue. The wall is very oblique so that she must bend far forward to sit on the toilet and even then she feels the wall against her back.

ii. She goes for a journey but leaves one day later than foreseen because she joined an organized night walk just the night before. So, on the first day of her journey she is very tired.

iii. Her mother is tired because she has to welcome and serve all relatives and acquaintances in her café after the funeral of an aunt. This is very tiring for her mother, especially because she is obliged to talk with everyone.

Discussion:

Medorrhinum was chosen because it fits the physical and the psychical dream picture:

i. Physical: Redness around the anus.
ii. Psychical: The sycotic state usually is compared with the picture of a blown up frog. This means that exaggeration and also boasting which refer to an Ego weakness.

Dreaming of a night walk refers to the keynote of Medorrhinum: 'amelioration during the night' and refers moreover to the sycotic theme 'tendency to exaggerate'.

The bending forward in the first dream is the contrary of what is known as a peculiar of Medorrhinum, 'Constipation, bending backward ameliorates', but here it is a kind of exaggeration.

In the last dream her mother felt obliged to talk to everybody. This suggests that she had no time for herself or to be conscious of her own self. This is also a link to the Medorrhinum symptom 'fear of opinion of others' which reflects a want of self-confidence.

Prescription: Medorrhinum XMK, which cured her.

2. **Theme: Dismantling**

Case 2:

A 47-year-old dentist came to visit me because of his low dorsal back pain in the left side. During the physical examination I noticed that he was sweating abundantly on a single part, namely only at the lumbar region. There were no restrictions of movement. He himself felt generally better when he did some exercise in the open air.

He dreamt that he still has his former car which is worn-out. Before he leaves the car, he runs the engine, which then suddenly begins to make shocking movements accompanied by a lot of noise.

The medication I gave him was Silicea terra because of:

i. Back, perspiration, lumbar region (asaf., clem., hyos., naja, SIL)
ii. Generalities, exertion, physical, ameliorates.

I saw him again with common cold symptoms and diarrhoea alternating with constipation. He had a tender point at the right temporal region from where the pain radiated to the zygoma.

The dream, he had a few days ago was, he notices a heavy failure to the base of his dentist chair. To repair, he first has to dismantle carefully the complete base and then he assembles everything again in a 180° turned position.

Afterwards he made himself the reflection that he always had difficulties to get structure in everything what he does. He said that the profession of dentist did not fit him properly. He always was obsessed by his hobby 'music'. He played music himself and had moreover a very expensive music installation, which he had bought recently.

During the physical examination I again noticed the abundant sweating at the lumbar region.

Discussion:

The persisting abundant sweating was an indication that the remedy Silicea terra, given a week ago, could only act partially. Such an incomplete process is caused in most of the cases where there is blockage of the ancestral energy. Such a blockage can only be eliminated by the administration of a classic nosode.

Consequently Medorrhinum was administered to the patient and shortly afterwards all his symptoms disappeared.

Comment:

In this case, it would be wrong to administer Silicea terra again. From personal experience I know that this would not bring a fast and complete improvement.

The reason is that the 'awakened sycosis' in this case would block the healing process for a long time. Even if this 'awakened sycosis' in a later phase proceeds to an 'asleep' stage and even the complaints of the patient disappear after a long period of waiting, nevertheless the Silicea terra state of the patient would not have been treated completely.

This blockage would stay partially in an underlying miasmatic layer. That is why, during a next period of discomfort, Silicea terra symptoms would reappear again. Consequently, a Silicea terra state with periods of improvement and regression would persist and come back again and again.

On the contrary, if we at that (correct) moment, when the underlying miasmatic state is awakened, administer the appropriate nosode, we can break this impasse. So, it brings about a quick and complete healing, and frequently on the occasion of the next consultation a total evolution of the patient which mostly corresponds to a change of his individual remedy can be seen.

3. **Theme: Going into extremes**

Case 3:

A 37-year-old patient dreamt that some boys climb on a climbing frame. One of them is very agile. Then something curious happens. Once that agile boy is at the top, he throws himself down and dies there on the spot. The spectators are not distressed (because he wanted it himself).

Cases 4:

Another 18-year-old patient had a similar dream: In the presence of her aunt, her mother and the entire family, the news is been told that her uncle with his mistress at work had an accident and died. Nobody is distressed, not even his wife and her sister.

Discussion:

Medorrhinum is a remedy which fits to someone who goes into extremes, in emotions as in behaviour. Thereby, Medorrhinum goes from one extreme to the other (Vithoulkas).

So, the young person climbs very agile to the top of the climbing frame and suddenly throws himself down, not even thinking of the possible consequences. This extreme behaviour dismisses the spectators of compassion when something like that ends up fatally.

The same happens to the person, who keeps a mistress and had an accident. The fact that this person had also a mistress is a projection of **exaggerated and perverse interest in sex**, typically in a lot of Medorrhinum patients (cf.: Symptom: Dreams, grief, absent*).

Syphilitic miasm

1. Auto destruction, self denial (crucifixion).
2. Fear of infection, impending disease, of being incurable.
3. Dreams of own disease.

Illustration by a case of Syphilinum:

A 46-year-old asthma sufferer dreamt about an enormous big house wherein, when entering you can look from the ground floor till the truss of the roof. Then suddenly she is inside rooms and she wonders in which way she is entering. In those rooms there is plenty of old junk, paper, clothes, etc. Through a tiny staircase she climbs till the truss of the roof and enters into a small room with only a bed and a chair. Then, all of a sudden, she is downstairs again in a kind of kitchen with a complete chaotic design although not disorderly.

The house reminds her of a labyrinth with criss-cross oriented rooms. She wonders 'Is there anything normal in this house?' Suddenly she arrives in a magnificent living room in green-blue tones.

Symptoms and themes:

An enormous big house, but empty and without structure, refers again to the emptiness of the Ego-structure. On the other hand the big empty house refers also to the **emptiness inside** the **megalomaniac structure** related to the indicated remedy.

i. Chaos
ii. Absence of harmony: Rooms are criss-cross, mingled and disoriented.

Discussion:

A big empty house refers to the **emptiness of the personality** of Syphilinum. The colours in the living room refers to her previous remedy Alumina.

Conclusion: Syphilinum shows itself clearly in the dream and is indicated here to remove an ancestral blockage related to her chronic disease.

Cancer diathesis

As already mentioned in the chapter 'Miasms and their psychological background; the mean feature of the cancer diathesis is EMPTINESS (of the individual) by which the person is predisposed to idealism or materialism.

Also mentioned in that chapter is the opposite tendency of self-realization in the cancer diathesis.

Fear or delusion of having cancer* (Vannier, L., Les cancériniques et leur traitement homoeopatiques, Paris : G.Doin & Cie Editeurs, 1952).

By going through the symptoms of Carcinosinum we notice:

1. History of domination: Excessive parental control, demanding parents or partner. This is mostly a repeating pattern through the successive generations.

    So, the person carries too much responsibility at a younger age and develops a strong sense of duty. So, these young people act like adults and miss their adolescence.

2. i. Want of self-respect, Want of self-love: Carcinosinum people have a yielding disposition and are very accommodating by nature. They always efface one selves and cannot say 'no' to the demands of others. They emanate to be 'totally yours'. So, others direct their life (Magnesium muriaticum).

   ii. Want of self-esteem. Carcinosinum is fascinated by the power of nature which is the reverse of his insignificance.

    Carcinosinum is also impressed by and is dependent on order, discipline and structure, and has the inclination to check everything twice. This dependence fits to a person who lacks inner structure.

   iii. Want of ego and need of guidance: this is reflected by the symptom 'ailments from absence of father.

3. Dream from the proving: Looking for someone and failing to find that person (Tempelton W. Lees).

    This dream frequently occurs in already married people, having even children, who look in their dream for a life partner and fail to find that person.

    Interpretation: Those people looking for their animus or anima which they cannot find. This means that this part of their personality is underdeveloped. This dream refers also to their need to procreate.

4. **Dancing, desire for; rocking ameliorates:** They feel better when they are in a rhythmic motion because by this they approach more and more to their (inner) 'centre' of which they are estranged. Carcinosium people are romantic, not in real touch with reality.
5. **Desire to travel; Industrious:** Denying their own feelings.
6. **Reverence for supernatural forces** (by which the person gets a chill or becomes very emotional), like seeing thunderstorm with lightning, the take-off of an airplane, sportsman who breaks a record, etc.

Illustration with an example (from clinical practice):

An eight-year-old boy suffered from dyslexia and had to stay down a class.

His last medication was Lycopodium clavatum. Since that time he was more quiet and asked a lot less attention. But on the other hand he had anxious dreams. In one of those dreams he was attacked by black cats which bite-off his forefinger.

Also his mother noticed that he got a serious growth of hair at the lower limbs.

i. Symptom: Hair, lower limbs (Carcinosinum).
ii. Symbolism of the forefinger (index).

The forefinger refers to the Ego, the individual part of the conscious. **So, the absence of it, because the forefinger is eaten up, consequently refers to the 'absence of own ego - individuality' in the dreamer.**

This confirms the choice of Carcinosinum as an intermediary remedy (after Lycopodium clavatum). Moreover both remedies are known as great remedies to treat dyslexia.

Tubercular diathesis

A tubercular patient has much imagination and lives in a **world of fantasy** which is not really in touch with reality. For a tubercular patient the body feels like a cage, but by his imagination he can escape and travel everywhere.

This **desire to travel** is also known as a strong craving for freedom, which in fact is a desire to escape away from oneself.

The astral energy of a tubercular patient is far out of his body and all his energy is in his enlarged aura. In addition to all the dimensions, he feels enlarged so that he wants to **explore the borders** which can give rise to **sexual perversity**. This all needs a lot of energy which can exhaust the person.

Case of Tuberculinum:

A 14-year-old boy received seven weeks ago Cisplatina 6 LM, to take every day. During that period he felt very well but in the last days he had some new complaints which disturbed him a lot. His appetite was now diminished accompanied with a fullness at stomach. After every meal he had an urge to go to stool. He also had pain at the right nipple. Another problem, which disturbed him already for a long time, was that he felt himself inferior because he was the smallest member of his basketball team. However, even in winter, he was wearing only a T-shirt. He had two dreams at that period: He is busy 'snowboarding' and suddenly he loses the control during a jump. He takes his head in his hands to protect himself. Happily he lands well.

In another dream his father receives an U-shape candle which burns at both the sides as a reward because he is the best skier.

Discussion:

    Symptoms: Delusion of being not appreciated (plat.)

                       Generalities, warm agg.

                       Dreams, happy end (cisplat.)

    Theme: **Candle with burns at both ends.**

                       Heat, sensation of: wears only a T-shirt

These led to Tuberculinum bovinum (cf. Vithoulkas).

Directly after the patient took Tuberculinum, the energetic picture of the patient turned back to Cisplatina.

So, at that moment, it again indicated to repeat the fundamental remedy Cisplatina of that patient, which I administered once again in MK.

Follow-up: Some days later the mother called me to tell that her son was again in best condition. Now, more than a year later he had a growth spurt and had now the average height of his team members of the basketball team.

Chapter 7

Bowel Nosodes

Nosode is used to denote a homeopathic remedy prepared either from actual disease tissue or from disease-associated organisms, i.e. bacteria and viruses.

The stool culture in many chronic diseases shows a presence of non-lactose fermenting bacteria, the so-called 'Bowel nosodes'. They are not really nosodes because they are not morbid products of disease.

It was **Edward Bach** (1886-1936) who started investigation and discovered that certain intestinal germs belonging to non-lactose fermenting, gram negative, coli-typhoid group had close connection with chronic diseases. These germs were present in the intestines of 'all' persons, but they were found to be distinctly increased in persons who suffered from a chronic disease.

When there is no disease, the intestinal flora is in balance and the Bacillus coli performs a beneficial function. But any stress or disease upsets this balance of the intestinal flora and is followed by a change in the habit and the biochemistry of B. coli which may then be called as pathogenic. So, B. coli is the basic organism from which non-lactose fermenting 'bacilli' and 'cocci' originate.

First Bach used the bowel nosodes as injectable vaccine preparations from killed cultures of the organisms. Later, in 1919 he joined the London Homoeopathic Hospital as a house pathologist and bacteriologist and introduced the bowel nosodes in homeopathic practice by making potentialised preparations of the vaccine of killed organisms.

Dr **John Paterson** (1890-1955), a Scottish physician who had worked with Bach on the nosodes, continued the research after 1928. He grouped and typed the flora and by continous experiments and observations, he was able to detect more clear indications for each type and a definite relationship between certain homeopathic remedies and certain types of bowel flora (see, addendum : List of relationships).

Bach found that the bowel nosodes were closely associated with the symptoms of the 'psoric miasm'. Paterson went further and made some relations between certain bowel nosodes and certain 'chronic miasms'.

So, Paterson suggested a relation between Psora and most bacillary forms (Dysenteriae compound [Bach], Morgan gaertner [Paterson], Morgan pure [Paterson], Mutabile [Bach], Proteus [Bach]), between Sycosis and most diplococcal forms (Coccal co. [Bach] and Sycotic co. [Paterson]) and between Syphilis and Pseudo-psora and some different forms (Bacillus 7 [Paterson], Bacillus 10 [Paterson] and Gaertner [Bach]).

The energetic examination shows another classification:

1. Psoric : Coccal co. (Bach), Morgan gaertner (Paterson), Proteus (Bach)
2. Sycosis : Bacillus 10 (Paterson), Morgan pure (Paterson), Sycotic co. (Paterson)
3. Syphilitic : Gaertner (Bach)
4. Tubercular : Bacillus 7 (Paterson)
5. Cancer : Dysenteriae compound (Bach), Mutabile (Bach)

This means that an intercurrent use of bowel nosodes can act upon the hereditary layer, like the classic nosodes.

When they act on a hereditary layer, which does not include the psoric miasm, there is always a therapy localization (TL) at Conception Vessel 24 (CV 24).

So, the psoric bowel nosodes, Coccal co. (Bach), Morgan gaertner (Paterson) and Proteus (Bach), do not have the acupuncture point Conception Vessel 24 but have a TL on Governing Vessel-15.

The other bowel nosodes do not have a relation with the Governing Vessel, except Bacillus-7 (Paterson).

The data on bowel nosodes is mainly obtained through clinical experience. This means that a stool examination of chronic patients has been done before administering the simillimum. Afterwards the relation between actual known homeopathic remedies and the types of cultivated bacteria has been made. Also, some provings have been done by Thomas Dishingston with Dysenteriae (Bach).

J. Paterson recommended the following strategy to select the correct bowel nosode :

The choice of a bowel nosode for any case can be determined by a study of the clinical history and noting the remedies which have given the greatest, although not sustained, effect. Tabulate this list of remedies and compare it with the nosode list and associated remedies and choose the nosode which has the greatest number within this group. By energetic examination we can accurately determine the correct moment of administration.

When a patient needs a bowel nosode, he responds to the hand mode for bowel nosodes*. Then, by controlling the handmodes for each miasm combined by executing the specific muscle tests, the correct bowel nosode can be selected.

JUDGEMENT OF THE ACTION OF A BOWEL NOSODE

The action of a bowel nosode is almost identical to the action of classic nosodes. Either they move a hereditary layer, or they act as a complementary remedy.

J. Paterson mentions :

In many cases there may not be much apparent effect from the nosode, but it would seem that the given nosode in some manner had readjusted the case, because thereafter considerable benefit follows the previously given remedy without much effect. If there seems no apparent benefit from the nosode, do not be disappointed but repeat the remedy which had given the evidence of partial reaction before, and this time you can expect a more permanent action.

In my practice, there is never a starting with a bowel nosode. A bowel nosode acts mostly as a drainage for the waste products which, after administration of the simillimum are secreted into circulation and are being retained in the body by an energetic, hereditary barrier.

At the moment the bowel nosode is indicated, the patient mostly returns with symptoms, which belong to the remedy picture of the previously given remedy.

Mostly there is a short period of amelioration, and then the sickness starts again. The energetic examination points to prescribe a nosode and **not to repeat the previously given remedy**.

This fall back is due to the hereditary layer, coming from one of the known miasms or diatheses. This protraction of the disease annoys the patient at that moment, but it gives **opportunity to treat a deeper, normally hidden layer and to save him from some worse evil in the future.**

Also, the symptoms which indicate bowel nosodes are not kept apart, like we do with classic nosodes. That's because bowel nosodes are directly related with their associated homeopathic remedies.

This means that the simillimum and the bowel nosodes overlap each other perfectly, contrary to the use of a simillimum and an intermediately given classic nosode (see fig. 7.1). A classic nosode can even be administered as a fundamental remedy.

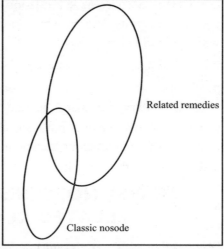

Fig. 7.1: Differentiation between classic nosodes and related remedies.

A bowel nosode does not stand as a fundamental remedy (remède de fond). That's why the bowel nosode is never repeated on the following prescription.

Either the previous constitutional remedy is repeated or a new remedy, that is complementary or related to the remedy administered before the bowel nosode is given.

Classic nosodes have more or less some individuality. But bowel nosodes have not. They lean against their related remedies which on the contrary have some identity.

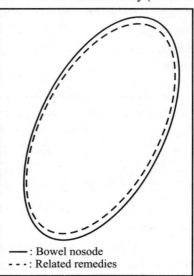

——: Bowel nosode
- - -: Related remedies

Fig. 7.2: Superposition of symptoms of bowel nosodes and related remedies.

This distinction is also reflected in the acupuncture points they use. Classic nosodes have a relation with the Conception Vessel and the Governing Vessel, which have both an individual course with own individual points.

Bowel nosodes do not have that relation (except for the non-psoric ones which have CV 24). Though they have a relation with other hereditary meridians, namely the extra (miscellaneous) channels, which does not have an individual course but use the points of different regular channels (meridians).

BOWEL NOSODES AND THEIR RELATED REMEDIES

Morgan-Gaertner (Paterson) : Ail.*, Alum.*, Ars.*, Atro.*, Bell.*, Calc., Caps.*, Caust.*, Cench.*, Cham.*, Chel., Chen-a., Chin.*, Cisplat.*, Cocc.*, Cupr-ar.*, Fl-ac.*, Gels.*, Graph., Hell., Hep., Ign.*, Indg.*, Kali-bi., Kali-c.*, Lac-c.*, Lach., LYC., Mag-c.*, Mag-m.*, Mag-p.*, Med.*, Merc-sul., Mez.*, Nat-m., Nux-m.*, Nux-v., Op.*, Phos.*, Phos-ti.*, Plb.*, Puls., Rumx.*, Sang., Sars.*, Sep., Sil., Sul-ac.*, Sulph., Syph.*, Tarax., Tub-a.*, Verat.*

Morgan Pure (Paterson) : Adeps-s.*, Alum., Ara-maca.*, Ars.*, Bar-c., Calc., Calc-f., Calc-s., Calc-sil., Caps.*, Carb-v., Carbn-s., Caust., Chel.*, Cor-r.*, Dig., Ferr-c., Graph., Gunp., Hep., Ign.*, Kali-bi., Kali-c., Kali-s., Lac-c.*, Lach.*, Lap-a., Lyc., Mag-c., Med., Nat-c., Nat-s., Nat-sil-f.*, Nux-v., Petr., Psor., Puls., Ratt-r-s.*, Rhus-t., Rumx.*, S.S.C [footnote], Sep., Sil., Spong.*, SULPH., Thuj., Tub., Vip.*, Vip-l-f.*

S.S.C. is associated by the name of Dr Henderson Patrick. The British Homoeopathic Journal : Potentized Drug Action on the Bowel Flora - by Dr John Paterson, lecture he read to the British Homoeopathic Society, March 5, 1936.

Bowel Nosodes

Proteus (Bach) : Alum.*, Am-m., Ambr.*, Aur-m., Apis, Bar-m., Borx., Calc-f.*, Calc-m., Chel.*, Chinin-ar.*, Chinin-s.*, Chol., Cinnb.*, Cisplat.*, Con., Crot-c.*, Crot-h.*, Cupr., Cycl.*, Equis-h.*, Ferr-i.*, Ferr-m., Ign., Kali-m., Lach.*, Lyc.*, Mag-c.*, Mag-f.*, Mag-m., Mag-p.*, Med.*, Mur-ac., NAT-M., Nux-v.*, Op.*, Phos.*, Rumx.*, Sec., Sep., Stann.*, Sul-i.*, Sulph.*

Mutabile (Bach) : Ars.*, Bry.*, Calc.*, Carc.*, Chel.*, Cupr-ar.*, Ferr-p., Kali-s., Lach.*, Mag-p.*, Phos.*, PULS., Rumx.*, Sil.*, Vip.*

Bacillus 7 (Paterson) : Am-i.*, Ars-i., Brom., Buddlda.*, Buth-a.*, Calc., Calc-f., Calc-i., Calc-p.*, Caust., Chel.*, Cinnb.*, Elaps*, Ferr-i., Grat.*, Hura*, Influ.*, IOD., Kali-bi., Kali-br., KALI-C., Kali-i., Kali-n., Lach.*, Lec.*, Lyc.*, Mag-i.*, Mag-m.*, Mag-p.*, Mag-s.*, Merc-i-f., Nat-i., Nux-v.*, Olnd.*, Onos.*, Oscilloc.*, Pall.*, Phos.*, Phos-ti.*, Rhus-t., Rumx.*, Sep.*, Sul-ac.*, Sul-i.*, Sulph.*, Tarent.*, Tub-a.*, Zinc-i.*

Bacillus 10 (Paterson) : Aral., Calc.*, Calc-p., Grat.*, Kali-bi., Lach.*, Mag-m.*, NAT-S., Puls.*, Sep., THUJ.

Gaertner (Bach) : Bell.*, Bothri-sg.*, Bry.*, Buteo-j.*, Calc-f., Calc-hp., Calc-p., Calc-sil., Cench.*, Cham.*, Chel.*, Con.*, Ferr-p., Fl-ac.*, Grat.*, Kali-n.*, Kali-p., Lach.*, Lec.*, Lyc.*, Mag-f.*, Mag-m.*, Merc-i-f.*, MERC-VIV., More-sp.*, Nat-m.*, Nat-n.*, Nat-p., Nat-s.*, Nat-sil., Nat-sil-f., Nux-v.*, Ox-ac.*, PHOS., Phos-ti.*, Phyt., Puls., Rad-br.*, Rhus-t.*, Rumx.*, Sep.*, SIL., Syph., Tarent.*, Tub., Zinc-p.

Dysenteriae Compound (Bach) : Ail.*, Anac., Arg-n., ARS., Cadm., Calc-ar.*, Carc.*, Chin., Chinin-ar., Cinnb.*, Cinnm.*, Graph.*, Kalm., Mag-c.*, Mag-m.*, Nicc.*, Nux-v., Puls., Staph.*, Sulph.*, Tub., Verat., Verat-v., Vip.*

Faecalis or Coccal co. (Bach) : Ail.*, Alum.*, Ambr.*, Ant-c.*, Apis*, Ars.*, Bapt.*, Bell.*, Bry.*, Calc.*, Cham.*, Chel.*, Coloc.*, Crot-h.*, Dulc.*, Elaps*, HEP.*, Hyos.*, Kali-c.*, Kalm.*, Lach.*, Lyc.*, Mag-f.*, Mag-s.*, Med.*, Merc-c.*, Nat-m.*, Petr.*, Psor.*, Rhus-v.*, Rumx.*, SEP., Sil.*, Staph.*, Stram.*, Sulph.*

Sycotic co (Paterson) : Ant-t., Aq-calc.*, Calc., Coloc.*, Ferr., Kali-bi., Lyc., Mag-m.*, Nat-m., Nat-s., Nit-ac., PULS., Rhus-t., Sep., Sil., Sulph., THUJ., TUB.-(bac.)

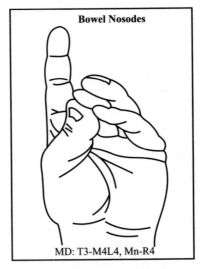

Fig. 7.3 Handmode of Bowel Nosodes

Energetic examination and clinical features of the bowel nosodes

All bowel nosodes have a positive reaction on the specific handmode of the bowel nosodes.

I. Morgan Pure (Paterson)

> **NB:** Paterson divided Morgan (Bach) into Morgan pure and Morgan-Gaertner.

Physiognomy and energetic examination :
1. Tender liver and gall-bladder.
2. Frequently an <u>open</u> ileocaecal valve can be diagnosed, which also has a TL at right outer ankle.

Muscle tests :
1. Weakness of the <u>left musculus sternocleidomastoideus</u> (relation with the stomach meridian), by which the head turns to the left side.
2. Weakness of the <u>neck extensor muscles</u> (relation with the stomach meridian).
3. Weakness of the <u>left or right musculus deltoideus medius</u> (relation with the lung meridian).
4. Weakness of the <u>left or right musculus pectoralis major - pars clavicularis</u>* (relation with the stomach meridian).
5. Weakness of the <u>left musculus piriformis</u> (relation with the circulation sex meridian).
6. Weakness of the <u>left or right musculus gracilis</u> (relation with the circulation sex meridian).
7. Weakness of the <u>left or right hamstring muscles</u> (relation with the large intestine meridian).
8. Weakness of the <u>left musculus quadratus lumborum</u> (relation with the large intestine meridian).

Morgan pure (Paterson) acts on the 'Sycotic miasm*' and has also the **same handmode as of Medorrhinum**.

This handmode does 'not' disappear when holding a bottle of Medorrhinum in the hand or on the navel.

The TL's on CV 24 and the right mastoid process are positive. There is a weakness of the <u>right musculus supraspinatus</u> when holding little finger upward with eyes closed, which refers to the weak ancestral energy.

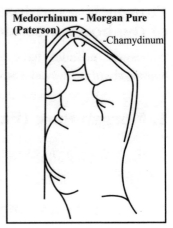

Fig. 7.4 : Handmode of Morgan Pure (Paterson) MD: IMRL/T against skin

Target organs: SKIN, integumentary tissue, lung and liver

Appearance and behaviour: Adapted to florid people with mostly a dark complexion. They are anxious and apprehensive about their state of heath.

Personal anamnesis: Weekly sick headache, post-zoster neuralgia, rheumatic fever, bronchitis each winter or <u>never well since pneumonia or bronchopneumonia</u>.

Keynote: Congestion.

Clinical observations :

1. Alopecia.
2. <u>Bilious headache</u>: <u>Congestive</u> headache and vertigo from high blood pressure.

3. Eruptions on margins of hair.
4. Cracks and eruptions behind the ears.
5. <u>Cracks at angles of nose</u> and at corners of mouth.
6. Blepharitis, styes and strabismus.
7. <u>Growth of hair on child's face</u>.
8. Very red lips.
9. Stiffness of tongue in the morning.
10. Recurrent tonsillitis with mucous out of cheesy pieces.
11. <u>Gall-stones</u>, cholecystitis.
12. Redness and moisture of bad odour at umbilicus (cf. Med.).
13. Piles.
14. Anal fissures.
15. <u>Constipation</u>.
16. Urethral caruncle.
17. Bartholinitis.
18. Athlete's foot.
19. Varicose eczema and ulcers.
20. Brittle nails.
21. Flat warts on hands.
22. Cracked skin on knuckles.
23. <u>Rheumatism</u>.
24. Waking at 5 a.m.
25. <u>Cracks</u>.
26. <u>Eczema</u> of the infant at teething stage or later.
27. Generalized fibrositis at chest wall, shoulders, cervical, dorsal, lumbar or sacro-iliac region.
28. Mongoloid.
29. Metastasis.
30. Alternating symptoms.
31. Vasculitis. Myocarditis

Energetic points:
1. At the left side: Bladder 13, 14, 44 and 48 and large intestine 8.
2. At the right side: In ninth intercostal space, on the posterior axillary line and Triple Warmer 4.

2. Morgan-Gaertner (Paterson)

> **NB:** Paterson divided Morgan (Bach) into Morgan pure and Morgan-Gaertner.

Physiognomy and energetic examination :
1. There is a contraction (trigger point) of the left musculus supraspinatus.
2. Right foot is warmer than the left.

Muscle tests :
1. Weakness of the <u>left or right musculus trapezius, pars ascendens</u> (relation with the spleen meridian), by which the scapula raises.
2. Weakness of the <u>left or right musculus serratus anterior</u> (relation with the lung meridian), by which the left scapula wings away from the thoracic cage (scapula alata) and it is difficult to raise the arm over 90°.
3. Weakness of the <u>left or right musculus pectoralis major - pars sternalis</u> (relation with the liver meridian).
4. Weakness of the <u>left or right musculus quadriceps femoris</u> (relation with the small intestine meridian).
5. Weakness of the <u>left or right musculus gluteus medius</u> (relation with the circulation sex meridian).

6. Weakness of the <u>left or right musculus gluteus maximus</u> (relation with the circulation sex meridian).
7. Weakness of the <u>left musculus quadratus lumborum</u> (relation with the large intestine meridian).

Morgan Gaertner (Paterson) acts on the 'Psoric miasm'. There is a positive TL on Governing Vessel 15. Also, a challenge with hands crossed above the pubis is positive in one way. The TL on CV 24 is negative.

Target organs: <u>Left colon</u> and urinary tract.

Appearance and behaviour: Adapted to irritable, impatient people, who often bite their nails. (Especially related to Lycopodium clavatum)

Personal anamnesis: <u>History of duodenal ulcer</u>, flatulent dyspepsia.

Clinical observations :

1. Alopecia areata.
2. Blepharitis, styes and cysts on lids.
3. Vitreous opacities and ulcer on cornea.
4. Boils in ear.
5. Red ears, yet cold to touch.
6. Otitis media and mastoiditis.
7. <u>Post-nasal catarrh</u>.
8. Sinusitis.
9. Polypus nose.
10. Fissures at angles of mouth.
11. Oedematous uvula.
12. Excessive eructations.

13. Gallstones, colic of left colon.
14. <u>Constipation with distended colon</u>.
15. Piles.
16. Anal fissures.
17. Prolapse of rectum.
18. Cystitis.
19. Nephritis and pyelitis.
20. Renal stones.
21. Tietze syndrome, left*.
22. Warty condition of nipples.
23. Heat of tip of (left) thumb*.
24. Warts on hands: Large, flat or jagged.
25. <u>Rheumatism</u>.
26. During sleep: Shrieks and uncovers feet.
27. Herpetic eruptions. Herpes zoster.
28. Urticaria. Psoriasis.

Energetic points: Governing Vessel 15 and Triple Warmer 12, at the left side.

3. Bacillus 10 (Paterson), also called Morgan 10

Physiognomy and energetic examination

1. Sensitivity of the sixth cervical nerve along the spine, on the left or right side.
2. Tenderness of coccyx.

Muscle tests:

1. Weakness of the <u>left musculus latissimus dorsi</u> (relation with the spleen meridian), which makes the left shoulder raise.

2. Weakness of the <u>left musculus deltoideus medius</u> (relation with the lung meridian).
3. Weakness of the <u>left or right musculus serratus anterior</u> (relation with the lung meridian), by which the heterolateral scapula wings away from the thoracic cage (scapula alata) and it is difficult to raise the arm over 90°.
4. Weakness of the <u>left or right musculus piriformis</u> (relation with the circulation sex meridian).
5. Weakness of the <u>left or left hamstring muscles</u> (relation with the large intestine meridian).
6. Weakness of the <u>left or right musculus soleus</u> (relation with the circulation sex meridian or triple warmer).

Bacillus 10 (Paterson) acts on the 'Sycotic miasm*'. The TL on CV 24 and the right mastoid process are positive.

Target organs: Lymphatic system and mucous membranes.

Appearance: Adapted to people especially of the 'hydrogenoid constitution'(= <u>sycotic miasm</u>), like Natrium sulphuricum and Thuja occidentalis.

Clinical observations:
1. Bores and picks in nose.
2. Crack in middle of lower lip.
3. Pruritus ani and vulvae.
4. Leucorrhoea of fishy odour.
5. Skin of groin is raw, dry and cracked.
6. Urethral caruncle.
7. ASTHMA associated with diarrhoea.
8. Panniculitis of chest wall.
9. Rheumatoid arthritis of left knee.
10. Warts on hands.
11. Lipoma: Fatty cysts in neck and lower ribs.

Energetic points: Conception Vessel 24 and right Mastoid process (cf. supra).

4. Proteus (Bach)

Energetic examination

Muscle tests:

1. Weakness of the left musculus sternocleidomastoideus (relation with the stomach meridian), by which the head is turned to the left.
2. Weakness of left musculus trapezius, pars ascendens (relation with the spleen meridian), by which the left scapula elevates, the dorsal spine becomes kyphotic and the left shoulder rolls forward.
3. Weakness of the right musculus pectoralis major - pars sternalis (relation with the liver meridian), by which the right shoulder raises and rotates forward.
4. Weakness of the left or right musculus iliacus or psoas (relation with the kidney meridian).
5. Weakness of the left or right musculus piriformis (relation with the circulation sex meridian).
6. Weakness of the left or right hamstring muscles (relation with the large intestine meridian).

Proteus (Bach) acts on the 'Psoric miasm'. There is a positive TL on Governing Vessel 15. Also, a challenge with hands crossed above the pubis is positive in one way. The TL on CV 24 is negative.

Target organs: PLASMA, central nervous system, sympathetic nervous system of capillary circulation (spasms), kidneys, liver and fibrous tissue of joints.

Appearance and behaviour: Adapted to nervous people of dark complexion and a thin, pale skin.

Proteus (Bach) is frequently associated with the muriatic remedies. They easily become irritable, especially on contradiction or if handled. Sometimes there is an outburst of violent temper with throwing things. When speaking, they can have sudden mental black-out.

Personal anamnesis: Effects from ultra-violet light (Natrium muriaticum), muscle cramps, ailments from 'a long period of nervous strain in business or family'(Ambra grisea and Lathyrus sativus) and divorces or separations in the family.

Keynote: Brain-storm.

Clinical observations:

1. Meningitis.
2. Ménière's disease.
3. Eyes are turned upward* (yin sanpaku).
4. Meibomian cysts.
5. Xanthelasma* (Chelidonium majus, Lycopodium clavatum and Sepia officinalis).
6. Cracks at corners of mouth.
7. Sudden haematemesis or melaena due to duodenal ulcer. Sometimes, there is even a perforation.
8. Frequent hiccough.
9. Oxyuris.
10. Angina pectoris and myocardial infarction. Sudden cardiac attacks at rest or while walking.
11. Bronchitis of old people with a lot of rattling mucous.
12. Prolapsed intervertebral disc with sciatica.

13. Rheumatism. Hammer toes. Cramps in dancers.
14. Deep fissures with marked induration on fingers and feet.
15. <u>Intermittent claudication</u> of lower limbs.
16. <u>Raynaud's disease</u>. Thrombophlebitis.
17. During sleep: Kicks head against the wall.
18. Angioneurotic oedema (Apis mellifica).
19. Herpetic eruptions at the mucocutaneous margins.
20. Symptoms appear with a degree of SUDDENNESS.

Energetic points: Governing Vessel 15 and Lung 6, bilaterally.

5. Mutabile (Bach)

Energetic examination

Muscle tests:

1. Weakness of the <u>left musculus deltoideus anterior</u> (relation with the gall-bladder meridian).
2. Weakness of the <u>left or right musculus psoas</u> (relation with the kidney).
3. Weakness of the <u>left or right musculus soleus</u> (relation with circulation sex meridian and triple warmer). This can create a forward lean due to poor posterior tibial support.

Mutabile (Bach) is associated with the 'Cancer diathesis*'. The TL on CV 24 and the convex line in the middle between the right ear and caudal extension of the sutura sagittalis under the linea nuchae suprema are positive.

There is a weakness of the <u>right m. supraspinatus, facing the palm to the body and with little finger upward with closed eyes</u>, which refers to a weak ancestral energy.

Target organs: Epithelial cells of skin, mucous membranes and circulation.

Appearance and behaviour: People who need Mutabile (Bach), resemble a lot to Pulsatilla nigricans (also indicated in Kalium sulphuricum and Ferrum phosphoricum patients).

Clinical observations:

1. Puffiness around the eyes.
2. Acute and chronic cystitis.
3. Painful, gouty nodosities on distal finger joints.
4. Puffy and blue hands and feet.
5. Skin has a sallow colour.
6. Perspiration during sleep.
7. Alternation of symptoms, e.g. skin eruptions alternating with asthma.
8. Malnutrition.

6. Bacillus 7 (Paterson)

Physiognomy and energetic examination:

1. Sensitivity of the fifth cervical nerve along the spine, on the left side.
2. Slow pulse rate, often with low blood pressure, due to myocardial weakness.

Muscle tests :

1. Weakness of the neck extensor muscles (relation with the stomach meridian).
2. Weakness of the left musculus supraspinatus (relation with the conception meridian).

3. Weakness of the right musculus subscapularis (relation with the heart meridian).
4. Weakness of the left or right musculus serratus anterior (relation with the lung meridian), by which the scapula wings away from the thoracic cage (scapula alata) on the weak side.
5. Weakness of the left musculus latissimus dorsi (relation with the spleen meridian).
6. Weakness of the left musculus piriformis (relation with the circulation sex meridian).
7. Weakness of the left or right hamstring muscles (relation with the large intestine meridian).

Bacillus 7 (Paterson) is associated with the 'Tubercular diathesis'. The TL on CV 24, the left mastoid process and the left Tuberculinum point situated on two inch distance from the anterior fontanelle are positive.

There is a weakness of the left m. supraspinatus, facing the palm to the body, which refers to a weak ancestral energy.

The **handmode of Tuberculinum** is positive but does not disappear when holding the different Tuberculinums.

Target organs: Neuro-muscular junction and fibrous tissue.

Appearance: Suits to tense, pale and tired people.

Keynote: Extreme mental and physical fatigue.

Bacillus 7 (Paterson) is especially associated with the halogens 'Bromine and Iodine', often in combination with Potassium.

Personal anamnesis: Tendency to syncope after sudden exertion.

Clinical observations :

1. Red ears, yet cold to touch*.
2. Angioneurotic oedema (eyes closed).
3. Thrombosis of central retinal vein.
4. Enteroptosis.
5. Sexuality : Premature senility.
6. Asthma. Bronchial catarrh (Kalium carbonicum).
7. Cracking of the cervical region on moving the head.
8. Cracks in palms of hands, knuckles and fingertips.
9. Cracking of joints.
10. Flat feet.
11. Ganglion.
12. Rheumatoid arthritis with nodules.
13. Dreams about euthanasia.
14. Faintness from long standing.
15. Excessive perspiration.

Energetic points: The whole course of the Governing Vessel is weakened.

Acupuncture points: Heart 2 on the right side, and Lung 6, bilaterally.

7. Gaertner (Bach)

Energetic examination

Muscle tests:

1. Weakness of the left musculus sternocleidomastoideus (relation with the stomach meridian), by which the head is turned to the left.

2. Weakness of the <u>right musculus subscapularis</u> (relation with the heart meridian).
3. Weakness of the <u>left or right musculus pectoralis major - pars sternalis</u> (relation with the liver meridian).
4. Weakness of the <u>left musculus latissimus dorsi</u> (relation with the spleen meridian).
5. Weakness of the <u>right musculus iliacus</u> (relation with the kidney meridian).
6. Weakness of the <u>left or right musculus tensor fasciae latae</u> (relation with the large intestine meridian).

Gaertner (Bach) is associated with the 'Syphilitic miasm' and has the same handmode as Syphilinum.

This handmode does 'not' disappear when holding a bottle of Syphilinum in the hand or on the navel.

The TL on CV 24 and the left mastoid process are positive. There is a weakness of the <u>left m. supraspinatus, with thumb upward with 'closed' eyes</u>, which refers to a weak ancestral energy.

Target organ : Nervous system (nerve cells).

Appearance and behaviour: Adapted to <u>nervous</u>, thin people with mostly a fair complexion, blue eyes, long <u>black eyelashes</u> and freckles.

Especially adapted to people in <u>extremes of life</u>, in nutritional disorders of children with poor developed musculature and in malignancy.

The patient is mostly nervous, has fidgety of hands and feet and bites nails. When angry, he is inclined to throw things. Physically undeveloped.

Keynote: Faulty nutrition.

Clinical observations:
1. Sausage-like swelling of upper eyelids just above the eyelashes.
2. Deep fissures on tongue.
3. Dry scaly eruption around the mouth.
4. Black teeth.
5. Coeliac disease. Vomiting from <u>ketosis</u>.
6. Threadworms.
7. Hydrocoele.
8. Bronchitis.
9. Circinate eruptions on sternum (Carcinosinum).
10. Fibrositis shoulder. Pes planus.
11. During sleep : Child does not want to sleep alone, wants to be beside the mother, wants light in the room, somnambulism.
12. <u>Ductless</u> glandular diseases.
13. Neurasthenia.
14. <u>Small-pox with extensive suppuration</u> and intestinal disorders.
15. Chicken-pox*.
16. Urticaria

Energetic point: Bladder 25, on the left side.

8. Dysenteriae compound (Bach)

> **Note:** Dysenteric co. contains Shigella dysenteriae, Shigella flexneri, Shigella boydii, Salmonella gallinarium and Salmonella typhysus

Energetic examination

Muscle tests:
1. Weakness of the right musculus supraspinatus, hand facing towards the body (relation with the conception meridian).
2. Weakness of the right musculus abdominis internus (relation with the small intestine meridian).
3. Weakness of the right musculus gluteus medius (relation with the circulation sex meridian).
4. Weakness of the left adductor-muscle group of the lower limb (relation with the circulation sex meridian).

Dysenteriae (Bach) is associated with the 'Cancer diathesis*'. The TL on CV 24 and the convex line in the middle between the right ear and caudal extension of the sutura sagittalis under the linea nuchae suprema are positive.

Also the **handmode of Carcinosinum** is positive.

Target organs: (Sympathetic) nervous system, capillary circulation, heart and duodenum.

Appearance and behaviour: Adapted to lean, fair people with dark hair, dark lashes and a pink, white skin. It's especially suitable for slow and insidious chronic states.

The patient has a fear of new doctors. He cannot keep still and stammers from excitement. Often, there are choreic movements of facial muscles or limbs, or there is a twitching of the eyelids. They desire to go from place to place, to go out, and then when out to get back home again.

Keynote: Anticipatory tension, like in Carcinosinum.

Clinical observations:

1. <u>Stammering from excitemen</u>.
2. Recurrent tonsillitis.
3. Hay fever
4. Thyrotoxicosis and enlarged thyroid.
5. <u>Congenital pyloric stenosis in babies</u> (Aethusa cynapium).
6. Duodenal ulcer, sometimes followed by pylorus induration.
7. Colitis.
8. Cramps of foot with adduction of toes.
9. Periostitis of the metatarsal joints.
10. Swelling of ankles and heels.
11. During sleep: Kicks bedclothes off and perspires on scalp.
12. Blisters between the fingers.
13. Flat warts on hands.
14. Urticaria.

Energetic points: Bladder 2, on the right side, and Triple Warmer 4, on the left or right side.

9. Sycotic co. (Paterson)

Physiognomy and energetic examination:
Sensitivity of the sixth cervical nerve along the spine, on the right side.

Muscle tests:

1. Weakness of the <u>left musculus latissimus dorsi</u> (relation with the spleen meridian), by which the left shoulder raises.
2. Weakness of the <u>left or right musculus teres minor</u> (relation with the triple warmer meridian).

3. Weakness of the <u>anterior ipsilateral cloacal</u>, especially on the left side.

Sycotic co. (Paterson) acts on the 'Sycotic miasm' (Paterson regarded it as a pre-tubercular remedy). The TL on CV 24 and the right mastoid process are positive.

Target organs : <u>Mucous and synovial membranes</u> and lymphoid tissues.

Appearance and behaviour: Adapted to sallow, pale (anaemic) and nervous subjects who have a greasy skin. They bite nails and have <u>puffiness, especially under the eyes</u>.

Personal anamnesis: Digestive difficulties in children, weekly sunday headache, tendency to syncope after sudden exertion, recurrent tonsillitis, albuminuria, mastectomia (malignancy), asthma and bronchitis.

Clinical observations:

1. <u>Alopecia</u>. Perspiration of scalp during sleep.
2. <u>Premature grey hair</u> (Syphilinum).
3. Blinking of eyelids.
4. Hairs on face and upper lip.
5. Twitching of facial muscles.
6. Cracks under ears and in angles of nose and mouth.
7. Hay fever. Vasomotor rhinorrhoea.
8. Lips are dry and cracked.
9. Persistent herpes of mouth.
10. Deep ulcers on tongue.
11. Wart on tongue.
12. Cheesy masses from tonsils.
13. Goitre. Torticollis.

14. Distended colon (Hirschsprung)
15. Prolapsus of rectum.
16. Perianal warts.
17. <u>Albuminuria</u>.
18. Pyelitis, cystitis and urethritis.
19. Vulvo-vaginitis and balanitis.
20. Cystic ovaries. Polypi uteri.
21. Patchy lung, sudden pain at base of right lung.
22. ASTHMA AND BRONCHITIS.
23. Impended respiration during coughing. Croupy cough.
24. Rheumatic fibrositis of neck, chest wall, shoulders and back.
25. <u>Arthritis of metacarpophalangeal joints</u>, especially of middle finger. Rheumatic nodule between metacarpal 2 and 3.
26. Brittle nails.
27. <u>Cracks</u> on fingertips, wrists and heels.
28. Pes planus.
29. During sleep: Perspiration especially on head, irritable cough at 2 a.m.
30. <u>Vesicular or varicellar type of eruptions</u> on face or body. Chicken-pox.
31. Foot and Mouth Disease (to be used especially as a prophylactic remedy).
32. Warts on mucocutaneous surfaces.

Energetic points: Lung 3, left and Large Intestine 6, right

10. Faecalis (Bach) (Coccal co.)

Physiognomy and energetic examination:

There is a contraction (trigger point) of the left musculus supraspinatus.

Muscle tests:
1. Weakness of the right musculus supraspinatus (relation with the Conception Vessel meridian).
2. Weakness of left or right musculus infraspinatus (relation with the triple warmer meridian).
3. Weakness of the left musculus serratus anterior (relation with the lung meridian), by which the scapula wings away from the thoracic cage (scapula alata) and it is difficult to raise the arm over 90°.
4. Weakness of the left or right musculus subscapularis (relation with the heart meridian).
5. Weakness of the left or right musculus tensor fasciae latae (relation with the large intestine meridian).
6. Weakness of the left or right musculus piriformis (relation with the circulation sex meridian).
7. Weakness of the right hamstring muscles (relation with the large intestine meridian.

Faecalis (Bach) acts on the 'Psoric miasm*'. There is a positive TL on Governing Vessel 15. Also, a challenge with hands crossed above the pubis is positive in one way. The ancestral hereditary energy is not affected though there is a weakness of the right m. supraspinatus. TL on CV 24 is negative.

Clinical observations:
1. Cellulitis and sinusitis (maxillaris).
2. Lymphangitis and recurrent boils.
3. Rheumatic fever.
4. Septic conditions and boils.
5. Streptococcal infection.

Energetic points: Governing Vessel 15, Triple Warmer 5, on the right side, and Stomach 12, on the left side.

Relation between muscle tests and bowel nosodes, in the direction from homeopathic remedy to weakened muscle

NB: When the same remedy is marked as well at the left or right side, it is only found clinically at one side. (E.C.) : tested with eyes closed.

(Tested with eyes open in right-handed persons)

Adductors:
 left : Dys.
 right :
Anterior ipsilateral cloacal : Syc.
Deltoideus anterior:
 left : Mut.
 right :
Deltoideus medius:
 left : Bacls-10, Morg-p.
 right : Morg-p.
Gluteus maximus:
 left : Morg-g.
 right : Morg-g.
Gluteus medius:
 left : Morg-g.
 right : Dys., Morg-g.
Gracilis:
 left : Morg-p.
 right : Morg-p.

Hamstrings:
    left : Bacls-7, Bacls-10, Morg-p., Prot.
    right : Bacls-7, Coccal, Morg-p., Prot.
Iliacus:
    left : Prot.
    right : Gaert., Prot.
Infraspinatus:
    left : Coccal
    right : Coccal
Latissimus dorsi:
    left : Bacls-7, Bacls-10, Gaert., Syc.
    right :
Neck-extensors: Bacls-7, Morg-p.
Neck-flexors, medial : Morg-p.
Neck-flexors, m. Sternocleidomastoideus:
    left : Gaert., Morg-p., Prot.
    right :
Obliquuus abdominis internus:
    left : Dys.
    right : Dys.
Pectoralis major - pars clavicularis:
    left : Morg-p.
    right : Morg-p.
Pectoralis major - pars sternalis:
    left : Gaert., Morg-p.
    right : Gaert., Morg-p., Prot.
Piriformis:
    left : Bacls-7, Bacls-10, Coccal, Morg-p., Prot.
    right : Bacls-7, Coccal, Prot.

Psoas:
    left : Mut., Prot.
    right : Mut., Prot.
Quadratus lumborum:
    left : Morg-g., Morg-p.
    right :
Quadriceps femoris:
    left : Morg-g.
    right : Morg-g.
Serratus anterior:
    left : Bacls-7, Bacls-10, Coccal, Morg-g.
    right : Bacls-7, Bacls-10, Morg-g.
Soleus:
    left : Bacls-10, Mut.
    right : Bacls-10, Mut.
Subscapularis, hand near chest:
    left : Coccal
    right : Bacls-7, Coccal, Gaert.
Supraspinatus, hand facing toward the body:
    left : Bacls-7
    right : Coccal, Dys., Mut. (E.C.)
Supraspinatus, little finger upward:
    left :
    right : Morg-p. (E.C.), Mut. (E.C.)
Supraspinatus, thumb upward:
    left : Gaert. (E.C.)
    right :
Tensor fasciae latae:
    left : Coccal, Gaert.
    right : Coccal, Gaert.

Teres minor:
    left : Syc.
    right : Syc.
Trapezius, lower:
    left : Morg-g., Prot.
    right : Morg-g.

Chapter 8

Psora and Nosodes

The psoric miasm or the internal itch-disease is considered by Hahnemann as the basic miasm, the source of every chronic disease, which expresses itself in the form of a skin eruption. The basic disorder is an inability to assimilate, which results in **deficiency syndromes** and stagnation. This imbalance of health manifests itself through functional disturbances, hypersensitivity of all sorts and neurotic expressions.

The nosodes which are related to the psoric miasm are:

1. Faecalis (Bach) or Coccal co. (Bach)
2. Morgan gaertner (Paterson).
3. Proteus (Bach).
4. Psorinum.

The energetic examination reveals a **Psoric point** (TL) on **Governing Vessel 15** for all of them*. This point (GV 15) is called the 'Sympathetic Master Point', which is situated between the atlas and the axis. In acupuncture this point has a general exciting and toning property by acting on the arteriomuscular vessels. This property is contrary to the stagnation, which is typical for psora. (This point is also a TL for Cuprum arsenicosum and Rumex crispus)

The main classic nosodes (exception of Psorinum) and the other bowel nosodes by exception of Faecalis (Bach), Morgan- gaertner

(Paterson) and Proteus (Bach) have, as I already mentioned, a specific relation with **heredity. This is reflected by a disturbance** of the conception and / or the governing channel. Their energetic points are independent from those of the 12 regular channels.

Also the psoric miasm acts on the ancestral energy, through the six other extra (miscellaneous) channels. Most of their energetic points belong to those of the 12 regular channels.

These extra (miscellaneous) channels are:

1. The **Chong Channel** : Coccal co. (Bach) (f. or m.), Morgan gaertner (Paterson) (f. or m.), Proteus (Bach) (f. or m.), Psorinum (f. or m.).
   TL at the medial transition of nose and upper lip.
2. The **Dai Channel** : Coccal co. (Bach) (m.), Morgan gaertner (Paterson) (f. or m.), Proteus (Bach) (m.), Psorinum (f.).
   TL at waist, bilaterally.
3. The **Yangqiao Channel** : Coccal co. (Bach) (m.), Morgan gaertner (Paterson) (m.), Proteus (Bach) (f.), Psorinum (f.).
   TL at Stomach 3, which is situated at the level of the lower border of the ala nasi, on the lateral side of the nasolabial groove, bilaterally.
4. The **Yinqiao Channel** : Coccal co. (Bach) (f. or m.), Morgan gaertner (Paterson) (f. or m.), Proteus (Bach) (f), Psorinum (f. or m.).
   TL at Bladder 1, which is situated 0,1 cm superior to the inner canthus, bilaterally.
5. The **Yangwei Channel** : Coccal co. (Bach) (m.), Morgan gaertner (Paterson) (m.), Psorinum (f. and m.).
   TL on Gall Bladder 14, which is situated on the forehead , 1 cm above the midpoint of the eyebrow, bilaterally.

6. The **Yinwei Channel** : Coccal co. (Bach) (f.), Morgan gaertner (Paterson) (f. or m.), Proteus (Bach) (m.), Psorinum (f. or m.).

TL at Kidney 9, which is situated on the medio-dorsal side of the leg at the lower end of the belly of the musculus gastrocnemius, five cm above the medial malleolus, bilaterally.

Till now I found some relations between these extra-channels and the anti-psoric nosodes, as mentioned above. Probably, each of these nosodes can disturb each one of these extra-channels. Mostly there is only one extra-channel disturbed when an anti-psoric nosode must be administered.

(f.) : Heredity from father's side.

(m.) : Heredity from mother's side. (cf. p. 55)

ENERGETIC SCREENING OF THE PSORIC NOSODES BY THEIR ENERGETIC POINTS

1. Faecalis: See chapter Bowel nosodes.

2. Morgan gaertner: See, chapter Bowel nosodes.

3. Proteus: See, chapter Bowel nosodes.

4. Psorinum

1. Muscle tests:
i. Contraction of the left musculus quadratus lumborum.
ii. Weakness of the right musculus quadriceps femoris.

iii. Weakness of the left musculus latissimus dorsi.
iv. Weakness of the left (sometimes the right) musculus rhomboideus.

2. Energetic points (Therapy localization):

i. Acupuncture points: Triple Warmer 4, left, can be used as W.P.; Triple Warmer 14, bilaterally; Governing Vessel 15; Bladder 49, right; Bladder 52, left; Spleen 7, left and Large intestine 14.

ii. Other Psorinum points are situated:
   a. At the cleft of the chin.
   b. On the convex line in the middle between the right ear and the sutura sagittalis, right above (2 cm) the upper implantation of the ear.
   c. Just above the protuberence occipitalis.

iii. Psorinum handmode: T3-14, OMR, -L. (See fig. 8.1)

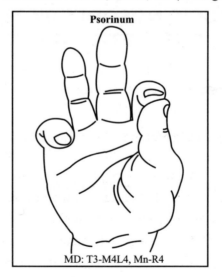

Fig. 8.1 Psorinum handmode

WORK SKELETON TO IDENTIFY THE SPECIFIC NOSODE

1. On condition that there is a change by applying:
   And/or
   i. TL on CV 24.
   ii. TL on GV 15.
   iii. Handmode bowel nosodes.
2. **Possibilities:**
   i. CV 24 and handmode bowel nosodes are negative, yet GV 15 is positive. We look for an anti-psoric nosode, Psorinum :
      a. Handmode 'Psorinum'.
      b. Muscle tests :
         - Weak left or right m. rhomboideus
         - Weak left m. latissimus dorsi
         - Weak right m. quadriceps femoris
   ii. CV 24 negative and handmode bowel nosodes positive. We look for an anti-psoric bowel nosode (NB: also GV 15 is positive):
      a. Coccal co. (Bach) :
         - Weak right m. supraspinatus
         - Weak **left or right m. infraspinatus**
         - Weak left or right m. subscapularis
         - Weak left or right m. tensor fasciae latae
      b. Morgan gaertner (Paterson) :
         - Weak left or right gluteus medius
         - Weak **left or right m. quadriceps (rectus) femoris**
         - Weak **left or right m. gluteus maximus**

c. Proteus (Bach) :
- Weak left m. sternocleidomastoideus
- Weak left or right m. psoas or iliacus

iii. CV 24 positive and handmode bowel nosodes negative. So, it is one of the non-anti-psoric classic nosodes (**NB:** GV 15 is negative):

    a. Carcinosinum : **Handmode 'Carcinosinum'**.
        Specific muscle tests : Left m. deltoideus anterior.

    b. Medorrhinum : **Handmode 'Medorrhinum'**.
        Specific muscle tests : Left m. latissimus dorsi.

    c. Syphilinum : **Handmode 'Syphilinum'**.
        Specific muscle tests : Right m. latissimus dorsi.

    d. Tuberculinum : **Handmode 'Tuberculinum'**.
        Specific muscle tests :

            bac. : right m. coracobrachialis (E.C.)
                      right m. teres major (E.C.)

            tub. : left m. supraspinatus, thumb upward (E.C.)
                      right m. coracobrachialis

            tub-a.: left m. teres major (E.C.)

            tub-d. : right m. serratus anterior
                      left m. deltoideus medius

            tub-k.: left or right m. deltoideus medius (E.C.)
                      left or right m. serratus anterior (E.C.)

            tub-m. : left m. supraspinatus

            tub-r. : right m. teres major (E.C.)

            tub-sp.: left or right m. serratus anterior (E.C.)
                      left or right m. coracobrachialis (E.C.)

Psora and Nosodes 169

iv. CV 24 positive and handmode bowel nosodes positive. So, it is one of the non-anti-psoric bowel nosodes (**NB:** GV 15 is negative):
   a. Cancer diathesis :
      • Dysenteriae compound (Bach): **Handmode of 'Carcinosinum'**
         Weak right m. supraspinatus
         Weak left adductor-muscles
      • Mutabile (Bach): **Weak left m. deltoideus anterior**
         Weak left or right psoas
   b. Sycotic miasm :
      • Bacillus 10 (Paterson): Weak right m. serratus anterior
         Weak left or right m. soleus
      • Morgan pure (Paterson): **Handmode of 'Medorrhinum'**
         <u>**Weak right m. supraspinatus, little finger upward (E.C.)**</u>
         Weak neck-extensors
         <u>**Weak left or right m. pectoralis major - pars clavicularis**</u>
         Weak left or right m. gracilis
         Weak left or right hamstrings
      • Sycotic co. (Paterson): **Weak left or right m. teres minor**
         Anterior ipsilateral cloacal
   c. Syphilitic miasm :
      • Gaertner (Bach): <u>**Handmode of 'Syphilinum'**</u>
         <u>**Weak left m. supraspinatus, thumb upward (E.C.)**</u>
         Weak right m. iliacus

d. Tubercular diathesis :
   - Bacillus 7 (Paterson): **Handmode of 'Tuberculinum'**
     Weak medial neck-flexors
     Weak left m. supraspinatus

Chapter 9

What Happens when the Interaction between the Individual Remedy and the Nosode Starts

What happens when a nosode is prescribed as a 'single' individual remedy (covering also the miasmatic background)

When an individual is subjected to a long-lasting stress, and when this stress is increasing more and more, it lessens the strength of the individual energy of the person, so that the hidden ancestral influences come up.

This ancestral energy sometimes becomes visible by the appearance of some nosodal symptoms, but in most of the cases there is nearly no symptom to perceive because ancestral nosodes do not have much individuality. That's why it is difficult to recognize those nosodes. **So, it is very important to think about them when there is a wasting of the individual expression and creativity in a patient. People who need a nosode have a weak personality.**

Mostly the personality which belongs to each of these nosodes is a **reflection**, as if by a mirror, **of the habits or the surroundings**.

So, a Carcinosinum patient is very tidy, conscientious about trifles and demanding. A Medorrhinum patient is very anxious concerning what will happen in the future and about his health. A Psorinum patient is introverted and pessimistic (feels separated and doomed) and has an unreasonable fright and fear of everything. A Syphilinum patient has the delusion of being dirty and the fear of becoming contaminated so that he frequently washes his hands. A Tuberculinum patient lives **like a candle which burns at both ends** because he has the sensation that the life is very short and he has to live very intensely now.

What happens when the individual remedy is complemented (directly) by a nosode which acts on an ancestral layer

In these cases the nosode acts as a miasmatical closure of the individual treatment:

1. In most of the cases I give the individual remedy in a Korsakov potency followed directly by the administration of the appropriate nosode.
2. Another possibility is when at the end of daily intake of a LM potency the patient comes back in a quite healthy state and I have to finish this treatment with a nosode, which is mostly Psorinum.

Just after the administration of the simillimum, we get an access to a hidden weakened ancestral layer. It is as if an ancestral weakness is drawn up to the surface by the immediate action of the simillimum.

This awakened ancestral weakness is linked to the astral or emotional load of some ancestors, e.g. a hereditary emotion or stress of one of the parents, grandparents or some other relatives (see Chapter 'Ancestral energy').

That is why the individual energy of a person is attracted at the moment of the incarnation to a certain couple of future parents, because the individual energy of that person in its pre-embryonic state fits with their astral or emotional ancestral load. So, just after the administration of the simillimum, it is as if a special layer of the ancestral energy is awakened **for a short period of time**.

At that moment we as homeopath get the opportunity to make a correction of this ancestral layer by giving a remedy which acts on the ancestral energy, namely a nosode. The action of this appropriate nosode can somewhat be compared with Family Constellations of Bert Hellinger on an individual.

Frequently in this short period, when a nosode would be indicated, we notice, especially in the dreams of the patient, themes of tensions in the family, which refers to the astral/emotional load of this ancestral layer (We can also see these themes during the intake of a remedy in LM potency if its action is finished by the intake of an appropriate nosode, mostly Psorinum).

So, when the affected ancestral energy is healed, the individual is cured from that ancestral astral/emotional blockage and its energy linked to a specific homeopathic remedy in which the individual was stuck. Consequently that individual can now develop more freely his own life and that is why his following remedy probably changes.

The common schooled classical homeopath normally does not give a nosode after the administration of the simillimum and mostly interprets the ancestral blockage, which rises up, as a homeopathic aggravation, but which is not. Luckily this kind of aggravation goes by after sometime (because the awakened ancestral energy goes to sleep again), and then the patient again reacts well on the same remedy (simillimum), which in the course of his treatment returns frequently during a long period of time.

So, if we do not administer that appropriate nosode, the individual energy gets stuck again in the same former energetic pattern and consequently the same remedy has to be repeated again and again for some period of time.

That is why classical homeopaths think that a remedy can only be considered as the simillimum of the patient, if that remedy has a curative effect for a long period of time. This means mostly that the remedy has to be repeated many times to obtain that effect.

On the other hand by giving the connected appropriate nosode, some correction of the ancestral energy takes place followed by a deep and long-term effect on the health of the person in all levels.

Chapter 10

Isopathic Nosodes

MONERA AND YEASTS

Monera are bacteria and viruses.

Yeasts belong to the kingdom of fungi.

Characteristics of Monera (according to Frans Vermeulen)

1. Invasiveness
2. Toxigenicity
3. Fast reproduction
4. Contagion
5. Communication
6. Colonisation
7. Strategy

Monera needs another organism to procreate themselves. So, similar to the Monera, the patient who needs a Monera remedy needs to know everything about the other in order to 'enter into'.

Characteristics of Yeasts

1. Aggression.
2. Invasiveness which is associated with death and transformation. Fungi take possession of the body and bring death.

3. Colonisation
4. Communication

The fungus body, the mycelium consists of a real network.

When to use isopathic nosodes (Monera and Yeasts)

1. We know from the famous homeopaths H.J. Allen, J.H. Clarke and D. Foubister that there is a possibility of administrating a specific mycotic, viral or bacterial agent in an energetic potency when the patient tells that he is never well since he suffered from a specific disease.
2. Experience also shows of this possibility when a case is blocked, especially after the adminstration of a correct simillimum.[1] This is very similar to the way nosodes were indicated by the former generations of homeopath.
3. It is proved that slumbering viruses and bacterias play a role in a large number of chronic diseases and syndromes as fibromyalgia, chronic fatigue syndrome, mutiple sclerosis, warts, allergy, emotional disturbances and various neurological disorders.
    i. In my experience it is mostly the need of an agent of viral or bacterial origin which blocks a case and which has to be administrated in a high dynamisation, once. Mostly it has to be directly followed again by the re-intake of the blocked simillimum, which must be reactivated.

---

1. When after the intake of a correct remedy, initially a short-lived recovery occurs which is then followed directly by a quick relapse, the cause of this is mostly the coming to surface of a hidden ancestral blockage or a blockage caused by an inherent bacterial, viral or mycotic agent.

    In most cases it is easy to recognise as the new symptoms and especially the dreams symptoms, appearing since the intake of the last prescribed remedy, still refers to this remedy. Sometimes, but not always, a specific symptom of the nosode to prescribe is also present. So, we see a prolonging of the state of the patient as before he took his simillimum.

Isopathic Nosodes

Some of them are very important to restore our weakened or damaged immune system.

Examples: The first exampe I want to give is of the group Influenzinum, Influezinum complex VSM, Mucococcinum and Oscillococcinum (and recently also A/H1N1) when the patient suffers from flu. In my experience this happens frequently in the autumn and winter shortly after the administration of the simillimum (and the nosode for ancestral correction, if the simillimum is not prescribed in a 50 millesimal potency). When it happens, the patient feels a lot better for some days and then again he gets flu symptoms. This is the moment when the patient has to come back and at that moment you will find one of these isopathic agents, mostly to be followed by Psorinum and sometimes even Medorrhinum which is related with flu. Directly after the administration of that mix, the former prescription has to be repeated, namely the simillimum (and the nosode for the ancestral correction).

Interpretation: The energy of the patient is taken up by the flu energy to make a spring cleaning of the body. The isopathic flu agent stimulates the good and quick development of the flu. Yet the flu has taken a lot of energy of the patient so that the intake of the simillimum has to be repeated directly after.

> **NB:** Sometimes it happens that, when there is much flu in the air, especially in patients with already some minor viral symptoms, one of the above mentioned isopathic agents is indicated directly after the intake of the simillimum (and the nosode for ancestral correction, if the simillimum is not prescribed in a 50 Millesimal potency). This can be energetically examined directly after administration of the simillimum and the associated nosode, when the patient closes the eyes for a while so that the energy of the simillimum and the nosode penetrates profoundly into the energetic body. If the patient now needs a surplus of one of these isopathic agents the energetic examination points to it.

The second example is that of the Epstein Barr virus, which often is used in a high potency in cases suffering from the Chronic Fatigue Syndrome. This isopathic remedy is frequently indicated when these cases come to a standstill during the classical homeopathic treatment. This standstill can be recognised by the absence of reaction in these patients on their simillimum, however the symptoms still refer to their simillimum.

Once the isopathic agent is administered, this administration has to be followed directly again by the re-intake of the blocked simillimum, which must be reactivated.

> **NB:** Clarke mentions the use of isopathic remedies as Coqueluchinum, Morbillinum, Parotidinum and Scarlatinum for the prevention and cure of whooping cough, measles, mumps and scarlet fever.

ii. Exceptionally the blockage is caused by the need of a mycotic agent. On the other hand a mycotic agent in a low dynamisation, e.g. 8, often is indicated in cases of some mycotic infection or after the intake of antibiotics. This is the moment the patient needs some mycotic remedy as a supplementary superficial remedy (in addition to the simillimum of the patient and the joined classic nosode).

We have the disposition of about thirty of mycotic remedies. Mostly this mycotic remedy has to be taken daily for some period of time, e.g. or some weeks. In that period it is recommended not to use cheese and sugar.

Practical confirmation: The ideal way to recognise the moment to administer an isopathic agent is by the energetic testing. The features of each of them are enumerated below. (The testing method can be read from the book: Physical Examinations and Observations in Homoeopathy, Degroote, F.)

ENERGETIC EXAMINATION, MUSCLE TESTS AND ENERGETIC FEATURES OF ISOPATHIC NOSODES

> **NB:** To be tested with eyes open (E.C.: If with eyes closed). All quoted muscles are weak if not mentioned explicitly. The specific quoted laterality refers to right-handed people.

Viral and Bacterial Agents

Common handmode: MD: T2I4R4, OM, -L (Léon Scheepers)

1. **Anthracinum (anthraci.):**
   i. m. biceps, left.
   ii. m. pectoralis major - pars clavicularis, left.
   iii. m. supraspinatus, tested with thumb upward, left.
   Energetic point: Lung 3, right.

2. **Bacteroides fragilis (bact-fr.) (code: 4614):**
   Sensitivity of the left nerve C3 along the spine.
   i. m. pectoralis major - pars sternalis, right.
   ii. m. gluteus maximus, right.
   iii. m. quadratus lumborum, left.
   iv. m. rhomboideus, right.

3. **Bartonella henselae (barto-h.) (code: 13921):**
   Sensitivity of the right nerve C3 along the spine.
   i. m. pectoralis major - pars sternalis, right.
   ii. m. pectoralis major - pars clavicularis, left.
   iii. m. triceps brachii, left.

4. **BCG :** MD of Tuberculinum.

5. **Borrelia burgdorferi (Lyme disease) (borre-b.):**
   Sensitivity of the left nerve C4 along the spine.
   i. m. supraspinatus, tested with little finger upward, right.
   ii. m. brachioradialis, left.
   iii. m. quadriceps femoris, left.
   iv. m. quadriceps femoris, left.
   v. m. gluteus maximus, left.
6. **Brucella melitensis:** See, Melitococcinum.
7. **Chlamydinum (chlam.):**
   MD of Medorrhinum acts on the sycotic miasm.
   Chlamydia resembles Medorrhinum. Verified symptoms of Chlamydia:
   - Headpain after ice cream (chlam-tr.)
   - Sterility in men and women
   - Flushes of heat at cervical region (chlam-tr.)
   - Oppression chest which ameliorates by rubbing and sitting erect (chlam-tr.)

   i. m. sternocleidomastoideus, left or right.
   ii. m. deltoideus anterior, left.
   iii. m.. latissimus dorsi, left.
   iv. m. supraspinatus, tested with little finger upward, left or right.
   v. m. infraspinatus, left.
   vi. m. pectoralis minor, left or right.
   vii. m. quadratum lumborum, left or right.
   viii. m. peroneus longus and brevis, left.
   ix. m. tensor fasciae latae, left or right.
   x. m. adductors, left.
   xi. Contralateral cloacal test.

Energetic points:
i. Conception Vessel 24, Bladder 15 (left).
ii. Lower margin of clavicula, 1 cm lateral from Ki 27, bilaterally.
iii. TL at right mastoid processus.
Dysfunction of the heart (sometimes solar) chakra.

8. **Clostridium perfringens (clostri-pf.) (code: 38063):**
   i. Hypertonic left m. rhomboideus.
   ii. Weakness of right m. infraspinatus.

9. **Colibacillinum (coli.):**
   - Personal history: Epididymis; Recurrent inflammations; Effects from oppression by a political regime
   - Swelling of upper eyelid at one side
   - Sensitive and swollen liver
   - Painful gallbladder
   - Eruptions about anus in infants
   - Pain kidney region, kidney stones
   - Swelling of joints of hands and feet
   - Chilliness immediately after eating (especially warm food*)

   i. m. rhomboideus, right.
   ii. m. psoas, left.
   iii. m. tensor fasciae latae, left.
   iv. m. gluteus maximus, right.

   Energetic points: Lung 2, right; Large Intestine 15, right; Stomach 10, left or right.

10. **Common cold virus (ccv-xyz.) (DNA rhinovirus) (code: 1358):**
    i. m. gluteus medius, left.
    ii. m. triceps brachii, left.
    iii. Hypertonic m. deltoideus medius and m. rhomboideus, on the left side.

11. **Cytomegalovirus (cytom-v.):**
    Chronic Fatigue syndrome.
    i. m. gluteus medius, left.
    ii. Hamstring muscles, left or right.
    iii. m. quadratus lumborum, left.
    iv. m. piriformis, left.
    v. m. tensor fasciae latae, left or right.

    Diaphragma point at Spheno-Temporal Line, right; which is situated perpendicularly above the external canal of ear.

12. **Diphtherotoxinum (diphtox.):**
    i. Hypertonic left m. anconeus.
    ii. m. pectoralis major - pars clavicularis, left.
    iii. m. supraspinatus, tested with little finger upward, left.

13. **Dysentery (dysentery)** (souche: Dolisos = probably only Shigella dysenteriae)

    NB: Dysentery is not equal to dys.

    Sensitivity of the left or right nerve C3 along the spine.
    i. m. supraspinatus, tested with thumb upward, left.
    ii. m. pectoralis minor, left or right.
    iii. m. trapezius - middle portion, left or right.
    iv. m. quadriceps femoris, left or right.
    v. m. popliteus, right.

14. **Eberthinum (eberth.) (Typhobacillinum):**
    i. m. supraspinatus, right.
    ii. m. deltoideus medius, right.
    iii. m. pectoralis minor, left.
    iv. m. infraspinatus, right.
    v. m. pectoralis major - pars sternalis, right.

vi. m. gluteus maximus, right.

15. **Enterococcinum (enteroc.)(code: 380(10)6):**
    - Pain transverse colon
    - Contraction of m. pectoralis major, pars clavicularis and pectoralis
        i. m. pterygoideus medialis, left
        ii. m. pronator teres, left
    Energetic point: N-UE-9, left (which is situated at middle of m. biceps brachii).

16. **Epstein-Barr / Pfeiffer (eps-b.):**

Epstein-Barr-virus/EBV causes infectious mononucleosis.

Chronic Fatigue syndrome.

Energetic picture by Léon Scheepers:
   i. m. supraspinatus, tested with little finger upward, right.
   ii. m. deltoideus medius, right.
   iii. m. trapezius - lower portion, right.

Energetic point: CV 24*

17. **Friedlander (mucot-kp.) (Klebsiella pneumoniae):**

NB: Friedlander is also a constituent of Mucococcinum.

Sensitivity of left nerve C3 along the spine.
   i. m. trapezius - lower portion, right.
   ii. m. latissimus dorsi, left or right.
   iii. m. rhomboideus, left or right.
   iv. m. serratus anterior, right.
   v. m. subscapularis, left or right.
   vi. m. gluteus maximus, right.
   vii. m. gluteus medius, left.

Energetic point: Large Intestine 15, left.

18. **Helicobacter pylori (helico-p.) (code: 22157):**
    Sensitivity of right nerve C2 along the spine.
    i.   m. supraspinatus, tested with little finger upward, right.
    ii. m. gluteus maximus, left.
    iii. m. sternocleidomastoideus, left.
    iv. m. latissimus dorsi, left.
    v.   m. quadriceps femoris, right.
    Energetic points: Right Bladder 15 and left Stomach 15.

19. **Hepatitis A (hepati-a-vc.) vaccinus:**
    Sensitivity of the left or right nerve C2 along the spine.
    i.   Hypertonic right m. trapezius, upper portion.
    ii. Hypertonic m. rhomboideus, left or right.
    iii. m. supraspinatus, tested with thumb upward, right.

20. **Hepatitis B (hepati-b-vc.) vaccinus:**
    Sensitivity of the right nerve C2 along the spine.
    i.   Hypertonic left m. trapezius, upper portion.
    ii. m. supraspinatus, tested with thumb upward, right.
    iii. m. rhomboideus, left.
    Dysfunction of the heart chakra.

21. **Hepatitis A & B (hepati-a&b-vc.):**
    Energetic point: Lung 3, right.

22. **Herpes genitalis (herp-g.):**
    Sensitivity of the left nervus C2 along the spine.
    i.   m. supraspinatus, tested with thumb upward, left.
    ii. m. peroneus tertius, left.
    Energetic point: N – CA – 10, left.

23. **Herpes simplex (herp-s.) nosode:**
    Sensitivity of the right nerve C2 along the spine.

Isopathic Nosodes

    i. m. supraspinatus, tested with little finger upward, left.
    ii. m. pectoralis major – pars sternalis, right.
    iii. m. quadriceps femoris, right.

    Energetic point: Circulation Sex 2, left.

24. **Hippozaeninum (hippoz.)** (virus-disease in horses, called Glanders or Farcy):

    Sensitivity of the right nerve C2 along the spine.
    Sensitivity of the left or right nerve C5 along the spine.

        i. m. deltoideus anterior, left.
        ii. m. deltoideus medius or posterior, left.
        iii. m. pectoralis major - pars sternalis, left or right.
        iv. m. teres minor, right.
        v. m. gluteus medius, right.
        vi. m. hamstrings, right.
        vii. m. peroneus tertius, left.

    Energetic point: Bladder 67, left or right.

25. **HIV (Aids nosode) (virionum):**

    MD of bowel nosodes

        i. m. supraspinatus, right.
        ii. m. supraspinatus, tested with little finger upward, right.
        iii. m. deltoideus medius, left.
        iv. m. trapezius - lower portion, left or right.
        v. m. subscapularis, left or right.
        vi. m. pectoralis major - pars clavicularis, right.
        vii. m. teres minor, right.
        viii. m. latissimus dorsi, right.
        ix. m. obliquus abdominis int. or ext., left or right.
        x. m. gluteus medius, left or right.

xi. m. gracilis, right.
xii. m. popliteus, left.
xiii. m. peroneus longus and brevis, left or right.

Energetic points: TL at left mastoid processus and CV-24.

26. **Influenzinum (influ.) vaccinus:**

    Influenzinum vaccinus acts especially on the sycotic miasm. Chill beginning at dorsal region and extending to and leaving by the nipples.

    i. m. supraspinatus, tested with little finger upward, left.
    ii. m. deltoideus medius, left.
    iii. m. latissimus dorsi, left.
    iv. m. pectoralis major - pars sternalis, left or right.
    v. m. trapezius - lower portion, left.
    vi. m. subscapularis, left or right.
    vii. m. gluteus medius, left or right.

    Energetic points: Bladder 22, right; Heart 2, bilateral; Gall Bladder 35, left or right; Stomach 8, left.

27. **Influenzinum complex (influ-co.) (VSM):**

    Streptococcus pyogenes 200K, Streptococcus pneumoniae 200K, Staphylococcinum 200K and Influenzinum 200K.

    i. Hypertonic m. pectoralis major - pars clavicularis.
    ii. TL at the left 7th intercostal space, on the median axillary line.

28. **Influenzinum pig flu (influ- A/H1N1)**

    Switching: 1/1; 1/1; 1/1; ...

    Hypertonic m. teres major on the right side

    Dysfunction of thyroid chakra.

    Energetic point: Lung 3, left.

29. **Lyssinum / Hydrophobinum (lyss.):**
    Sensitivity of the right nerve C2 along the spine.
    i. m. anconeus, left.
    ii. m. supraspinatus, right.
    iii. m. trapezius - upper portion, left.
    iv. m. tensor fasciae latae, left.

30. **Malaria nosode / officinalis (malar.) (code: 3174):**
    i. m. biceps brachii, left.
    ii. m. pectoralis major - pars sternalis, left.
    iii. m. iliacus, left.
    Energetic points: Lung 2, right; Spleen 9, left and Triple Warmer 12, right.

31. **Malandrinum (maland.):**
    Virus disease in horses, called as 'Grease'.
    Sensitivity of the left nerve C4 along the spine.
    i. m. deltoideus posterior, left.
    ii. m. serratus anterior , left.
    iii. m. coracobrachialis, left.
    iv. m. teres minor, right.
    v. m. psoas, right.
    vi. m. gluteus maximus, left.
    vii. m. quadriceps femoris, left.
    viii. m. tensor fasciae latae, left.
    ix. m. hamstrings, left.
    x. m. gracilis and adductors, right.

32. Melitococcinum (brucel.) Malta fever, Brucella melitensis, Brucellosis:

Melitococcinum acts on the tubercular diathesis.

i. m. supraspinatus, left or right.
ii. m. deltoideus anterior, left or right.
iii. m. teres minor, left.
iv. m. teres major, right.
v. m. trapezius - lower portion, left or right.
vi. m. hamstrings, left or right.
vii. m. tibialis anterior, left or right.
viii. m. adductors, right.
ix. m. gluteus medius, left or right.

Energetic points:

i. Bladder 2, right.
ii. Tuberculinum point, which is situated 2 cm from the anterior fontanelle, left; and also the MD of Tuberculinum.

33. Meningococcale vaccinum (meningoc-vc.):

i. m. coracobrachialis, left.
ii. m. sacrospinalis.
iii. m. trapezius - middle portion, left.

34. Micrococcus tetragenius (mucot-mt.) (code: 28323) :

NB: Micrococcus tetragenius is a constituent of Mucococcinum.

i. Hypertonic left m. sternocleidomastoideus.
ii. m. pectoralis major - pars sternalis, right.
iii. m. supraspinatus, tested with thumb upward, right.

Energetic points:

i. Lung 2, left.
ii. Lung 7, right.

35. **Molluscus contagiosum (molu.):**
    i. m. biceps, right.
    ii. m. abdominis obliqous internus, right.
    iii. m. rhomboideus, left.
36. **Morbillinum (morb.)** (isopathic nosode of measles):
    i. m. serratus anterior, left.
    ii. m. popliteus, left.
    Energetic point: Large Intestine 3, left or right.
37. **Mucococcinum (mucoc.) (Klebsiella pneumoniae, Brahamella catarrhalis, Micrococcus tetragenius and Influenzinum):**
    Sensitivity of the nerve C4, left or right.
    i. m. sternocleidomastoideus, left.
    ii. m. popliteus, left.
    iii. m. peroneus tertius, left.
    iv. m. teres major, right.
    Energetic points:
    i. Large Intestine 4, bilaterally.
    ii. Bladder 19, left.
38. **Mucotoxinum:** see, Friedlander (mucot-kp.) and Micrococcus tetragenius.
39. **Mycoplasma pneumoniae (mycopl-pn.):**
    Sensitivity of the right nerve C2 along the spine.
    i. m. latissimus dorsi, left.
    ii. m. gracilis, left.
40. **Oscillococcinum (oscilloc.):**

    NB: However it does not contain any viral or bacterial substance, it reacts to the viral and bacterial MD.

    i. m. deltoideus anterior, left.

ii. m. supraspinatus, right.

iii. m. rhomboideus, left.

When closing the eyes, the right m. psoas becomes contracted and the left m. supraspinatus, hand faced towards the body, becomes weak.

Energetic points:
i. Governing Vessel 5.
ii. Bladder 42, bilaterally. Bladder 51, bilaterally.

41. **Parapertussinum (parapert.) (code: 85(10)3):**
Sensitivity of the twelfth dorsal nerve, at the left side.
Hypertonic left musculus gluteus maximus.
– m. pectoralis major – pars sternalis, right

42. **Parotidinum / Ourlianum (parot.):**
MD: Chakra-evaluation (T4I4, TnM4, ORL) + Chakra (knee reflexes). Dysfunction of the solar chakra.
i. Neck extensors.
ii. m. biceps, right.
iii. m. peroneus longus and brevis, left.
Energetic point: Conception Vessel 20.

43. **Pertussinum /Coqueluchinum (pert.):**
Clinical observation: Coldness of back of feet during fever*.
i. m. latissimus dorsi, left or right.
ii. m. serratus anterior, left.
iii. m. trapezius - lower portion, left or right.
iv. m. gluteus maximus, left or right.
v. m. piriformis, left or right.

Energetic points:
  i. Right side: M-UE 48 and Small Intestine 11.
  ii. Left side: TW 14.

44. **Poliomylitidinum vaccinus sabinus (polio-vc-sn.):**
Sensitivity of the right nerve C3 along the spine.
  i. m. supraspinatus, right.
  ii. m. levator scapulae, right.
  iii. m. subscapularis, left.
  iv. m. pectoralis major - pars sternalis, right.
  v. m. quadratus lumborum, right.
  vi. m. gluteus maximus, left or right.
  vii. m. quadriceps femoris, right.
  viii. m. tensor fasciae latae, left.
  ix. m. popliteus, right.
  x. m. peroneus longus and brevis, right.

45. **Prevotella intermedia (prevo-im.) (code: 0372(10)5):**
Disease: gingivitis; rheumatic complaints*
  i. Hypersensitivity of the third left lumbar nerve (along the spine).
  ii. Contraction of the left musculus latissimus dorsi
  iii. Contraction of the right musculus pectoralis minor
  iv. Weakness of the right musculus peroneus longus & brevis

46. **Proteus mirabilis (prot-mir.):**

NB: Proteus mirabilis is not same as Proteus Bach, of which proteus mirabilis is probably a constituent.

  i. m. deltoideus medius, left.
  ii. m. rhomboideus, left or right.
  iii. m. quadratus lumborum, left or right.

Energetic points:
  i. M-BW-23, right.
  ii. Stomach 19, left or right.

47. **Pyrogenium (pyrog.):**
  i. Anterior ipsilateral cloacal test.
  ii. m. deltoideus medius, left.
  iii. m. gracilis, left or right.
  iv. m. rhomboideus, left.

Energetic points:
  i. Bladder 25.
  ii. Conception Vessel 5.
  iii. Lung 11.
  iv. Small Intestine 3.

48. **Rota virus (rota) (code: 1326):**
  i. m. deltoideus anterior, left.
  ii. m. quadratus lumborum, left.
  iii. m. obliquus abdominis internus, left.
  iv. m. tensor fasciae latae, left.

49. **RS - virus (rs-v.):**
Sensitivity of the left fifth lumbar nerve along the spine.
  i. m. supraspinatus, tested with little finger upward, right.
  ii. m. peroneus tertius, left/ (or in contraction).
  iii. m. infraspinatus, left or right.

Energetic point: Bladder 14, bilaterally.

50. **Scarlatininum (scarl.) (isopathic nosode of scarlet fever):**
  i. m. hamstring muscles, right.
  ii. m. gluteus maximus, right.
  iii. m. pectoralis major - pars clavicularis, right.

51. **Shigella (shigella-xyz.) (code: 295):**
    i. Hypertonic right m. pectoralis major - pars sternalis.
    ii. Hypotonic left adductor muscles.
    Energetic point: Kidney 24, right.
52. **Staphylococcinum (staphycoc.):**
    i. m. sternocleidomastoideus, left.
    ii. m. deltoideus posterior, left.
    iii. m. pectoralis minor, right.
    iv. m. teres major, left or right.
    v. m. teres minor, right.
    vi. m. latissimus dorsi, left or right.
    vii. m. quadratus lumborum, right.
53. **Staphylococcus aureus (staphyloc-a.):**
    Sensitivity of the left nerve C3 along the spine.
    i. m. teres minor, left or right.
    ii. m. latissimus dorsi, left.
    iii. m. pectoralis major - pars sternalis, left.
54. **Streptococcinum (streptoc.):**
    Sensitivity of the left or right nerve C3 along the spine. TL on the right spina iliaca posterior superior.
    Symptoms:
    Hearing illusions, crying for help, taste salty lips
    i. Hypertonic right m. quadratus lumborum.
    ii. m. sternocleidomastoideus, left.
    iii. m. supraspinatus, left or right.
    iv. m. pectoralis major - pars clavicularis, right.
    v. m. obliquus abdominis internus, left or right.
    vi. m. gluteus medius, left or right.
    vii. m. tensor fasciae latae, left or right.

Energetic point: Large Intestine 9, right.

Especially indicated in cases of chronic tonsillitis and sinusitis.

55. Tetanotoxinum (tetox.):
   i. m. supraspinatus, tested with little finger upward, right.
   ii. m. anconeus, left.
   iii. m. quadratus lumborum, left or right.
   iv. m. gluteus medius, left.
   v. m. gracilis, left.
   vi. m. tibialis anterior, right.

Energetic points: Bladder 3, left; Conception Vessel 18.

56. Toxoplasmosis nosode (toxo-g.):
   i. m. deltoideus anterior, right.
   ii. m. infraspinatus, left or right.
   iii. m. teres minor, left or right.
   iv. m. sacrospinalis - thoracal part.
   v. m. quadriceps femoris, left or right.
   vi. m. gracilis, right.

57. Ureaplasma genitalium (myco-gn.) (code: 32958):
Sensitivity of the left nerve C3 along the spine.
   i. Contraction of left m. pectoralis major - pars clavicularis.
   ii. Contraction of right m. quadriceps femoris.

58. Ureaplasma urealytica (urpl-ul.):
   i. m. subscapularis, right.
   ii. m. deltoideus anterior, left.
   iii. m. supraspinatus, tested with little finger upward, right.
   iv. m. teres major, left.

The left m. teres major is mostly hypotonic but can be also sometimes hypertonic.

Energetic points:
  i.   Conception Vessel 14.
  ii. Gall Bladder 23.
  iii. Heart 2, left.
  iv. Bladder 3, left.

59. **Vaccininum (vac.) (nosode from vaccine matter: cow pox):**
    Indicated in chicken pox, Herpes zoster, acute* and smallpox.
    Sensitivity of the left or right nerve C4 along the spine.
      i.   m. supraspinatus, left.
      ii. m. pectoralis major - pars sternalis, left or right.
      iii. m. pectoralis minor, right.
      iv. m. gluteus maximus, right.
    Energetic point: Bladder 50, right.

60. **Varicellinum (varic.) (isopathic nosode of chickenpox):**
    Indicated in chicken pox* and herpes zoster, acute*.
    Sensitivity of the left nerve C2 along the spine.
      i.   m. dupraspinatus, left or right.
      ii.   m. supraspinati, tested with little finger upward, tested together.
      iii. m. rhomboideus, left or right.
      iv.   m. teres minor, left.
      v.   m. pectoralis major – pars sternalis, left.
      vi.   m. obliquus abdominis internus or externus, left.
      vii. m. psoas, left or right.
      viii. m. gluteus maximus, right.
      ix.   m. gluteus medius, right.

x. m. tensor fasciae latae, left or right.
   xi. m. sartorius, left or right.
   Energetic points:
   i. Circulation Sex 2, right.
   ii. Large Intestine 5, right.
61. **Variolinum (vario.) (isopathic nosode made of lymph from a small pox pustule or a small pox extraction from the vesicle)**
   Indicated in chicken pox; herpes zoster, acute*; post-herpetic neuralgia and small pox.
   Sensitivity of the left sixth cervical nerve along the spine.
   i. m. latissimus dorsi, left or right.
   ii. m. subscapularis, left.
   iii. m. serratus anterior, left.
   iv. m. teres major, left.
   Energetic point: Bladder 24, left.
62. **Yellow fever vaccinum (yell-vc.):**
   i. m. quadratus lumborum, left.
   ii. m. sternocleidomastoideus, left.
   iii. m. teres major, left.
   iv. m. hamstring, left.

Mycotic Agents

Common handmode: MD: Fungi / Micro-mycotic germs, or T3-R4, -IML, or dorsal distal phalanges of IMR against skin.

1. **Actinomyces albus / Streptomyces albus (actin-a.):** Till now there is no energetic picture.
2. **Actinomyces citreus / Streptomyces citreus (actin-c.):**
   i. Pathology: Insufficiency of veins, varices, gastritis and gastric ulcers.

Isopathic Nosodes

ii. Energetic examination:
    CV 12   Left m. sternocleidomastoideus
    Li. 13, l. or r. Left m. latissimus dorsi
    St. 25, l. or r. Left m. quadratus lumborum
    CV 4   Left m. quadriceps femoris

3. **Actinomyces griseus / Streptomyces griseus (actin-g.):**
    i. Pathology: Vertigo, tinnitus, hardness of hearing in elderly people, otitis, catarrh of eustachian tube, leucorrhoea, vulvo-vaginitis and balanitis.
    ii. Energetic examination:
        CV 4   Left m. quadriceps femoris
        CV 14   Left m. subscapularis

4. **Actinomyces luteus (actin-l.):**
    i. Pathology: Till now there is no energetic picture.
    ii. Energetic examination:
        Bl. 3, l.   Left m. supraspinatus, tested with thumb upward
        Le 13   Left m. latissimus dorsi

5. **Aleurisma castellani (aclad.):**
    i. Pathology: Dysmenorrhoea, premenstrual syndrome (mastodynie) and mycosis of toe nail*.
    ii. Energetic examination:
        Li. 14, bil.   Right m. romboideus
        CV 3   Right m. peroneus tertius
        CV 12 (there is not a corresponding muscle till now)

6. **Aleurisma lugdunense / canis (aleur-l.):**
    i. Pathology: Acts on blood vessels causing arteriosclerosis and idiopathic hypertension, chronic pancreatitis, mental depression, neuro-vegetative dysfunction, spasmophily.

ii. Energetic examination:

Ha 2, l.

Li. 14

Bl. 3 (E.C.)   Right m. supraspinatus (thumb upward)- E.C.

7. **Aspergillus bronchialis (asperg-br.):**
   i. Pathology: Acute and chronic tracheo-bronchitis, flu, asthma, spasmodic nose-catarrh.
   ii. Energetic examination:

Ga. 25	Left or right m. iliacus or m. psoas
CV 3	Right m. peroneus longus and brevis and/or m. sacrospinalis
CV 12	Right m. brachioradialis
Lo. 5	

8. **Aspergillus flavus (asperg-fl.):** Till now there is no energetic picture.

9. **Aspergillus fumigatus (asperg-fu.):**
   i. Pathology: Acute and recurrent cystitis, chlamydia and other protozoa, infections of respiratory tract and lungs, flu, acute bronchitis, tuberculosis.
   ii. Energetic examination:

Lu. 1, bil.	Right m. serratus anterior
CV 17	Left m. gluteus medius
	Right adductor muscles

10. **Aspergillus niger (asperg-n.):**
    i. Pathology: Obesity, affections of prostate gland, nocturnal enuresis in children, thyroid affections, affections of the gastrointestinal tract, insufficiency of coronary arteries and heart.

ii. Energetic examination:

CV 12

CV 17   Left m. gluteus maximus

Right m. gluteus medius

Right adductor muscles

11. **Candida albicans / Monilia albicans (moni.):**
    i. Pathology: Kraurosis vulvae (lichen), leucorrhoea, vulvo-vaginitis, balanitis, intertrigo, ringworm, eczema of swimmers, cheilosis (erosion of corners of mouth in elderly people), psoriasis, dandruff, itch, black-coated and burning tongue, moniliasis, abdominal colic, recurrent rhino-pharyngitis, asthma, atopic eczema, hay-fever.
    ii. Mental picture:
        a. Delusion of being stupid.
        b. Anger and aggression, biting, destructiveness from suppressed emotions.
        c. Dreams of warfare, brutality, bombs, dead bodies, explosions, fire, murder, hell and rape.
    iii. Energetic examination:

    CV 3   Right or left m. peroneus tertius

    CV 12   Right or left m. subscapularis

    CV 17   Right or left m. gluteus maximus

    Li. 13, l.   Right or left m. latissimus dorsi

    Ga. Bl. 24, bil.   Right m. deltoideus anterior

12. **Cladosporium lugdunense (clados-l.):** Till now there is no energetic picture.
13. **Cladosporium metanigrum (clados-m.):**
    i. Pathology: Hepatitis, gastritis, gastric ulcers, dyskinetic

gall-bladder, chronic pancreatitis, arthrosis, rheumatoid arthritis and urticaria.

ii. Energetic examination:

CV 3	Left m. peroneus longus and brevis
CV 12	Left m. sternocleidomastoideus
Li 13, l.	Left m. latissimus dorsi
Ga. 24	Right m. popliteus
Bl. 37, l. or r.	

14. **Fusarium oxysporum (fus.):**
    i. Pathology: Infection of the urinary tract (acute and recurrent cystitis caused by coli, proteus, chlamydia, etc.), abdominal colic, infections of respiratory tract, flu, recurrent rhino-pharyngitis, acute bronchitis, otitis, catarrh of eustachian tube and rheumatoid arthritis.
    ii. Energetic examination:

CV 3	Left m. peroneus longus and brevis
CV 12	Left m. biceps
CV 17	Left m. gluteus maximus
Lu. 1, bil.	Left m. coracobrachialis
Ga. Bl. 24, bil.	

15. **Mucor mucedo (mucor):**
    i. Pathology: Arthrosis, rheumatoid arthritis, idiopathic hypertension*.
    ii. Symptom: seashore, lond stay at seashore am.
    iii. Energetic examination:

CV 3	Left m. peroneus tertius
CV 14	Left m. subscapularis
CV 17	Right m. gluteus maximus

St. 25, l.   left m. quadratus lumborum

Ha.1, r.

16. **Penicillium candidum (penic-can.):**
    i. Pathology: Acute and recurrent cystitis, infections of respiratory tract, flu, recurrent rhino-pharyngitis, acute bronchitis.
    ii. Energetic examination:

Lu. 1, bil.	Right m. rhomboideus
Li. 13	Left m. latissimus dorsi
Ga. Bl. 24	Left m. deltoideus anterior

17. **Penicillium caseicolum (penic-cas.):**
    i. Pathology: Constipation, abdominal colic, moniliasis.
    ii. Energetic examination:

    CV 12

    Sto. 3, l.

18. **Penicillium chrysogenum (penic-chr.):**
    i. Pathology: Paraodontitis, itch in ears, affections of the prostrate gland, red-spotted face.
    ii. Energetic examination:

CV 4	Right m. quadratus femoris
CV 14	Right m. sternocleidomastoideus
CV 17	Right m. gluteus medius
Li. 13, l.	Left m. triceps
Li. 14, bil.	Left m. rhomboideus

19. **Penicillium cyclopodium (peni-cy.):**
    i. Pathology: Arthrosis and rheumatoid arthritis.
    ii. Energetic examination:

CV 3	Right m. peroneus longus and brevis

CV 12	Left m. biceps
Li. 14, bil.	Right m. rhomboideus
L.I. 2, bil.	There is not a corresponding muscle till now

20. Penicillium expansum / glaucum (penic-e.):

i. Pathology: Mental depression and anxiety, CFS (weak adrenal glands), mental instability in children, enuresis nocturnae.

b. Energetic examination:

Bl. 3, l.	Right m. supraspinatus, tested with little finger upward
CV 4 (E.C.)	Left m. quadriceps femoris (E.C.)
CV12	There is not a corresponding muscle till now
Lu. 1, bil.	There is not a corresponding muscle till now

21. Penicillium griseum (penic-g.):

i. Pathology: Asthma.

ii. Energetic examination:

Ha. 2, l.	Left m. teres major
Li. 13	Left m. trapezius, lower portion

22. Penicillium notatum (penic-n.):

i. Pathology: Diarrhoea, atopic eczema, urticaria, hay-fever, recurrent rhinopharyngitis, chronic bronchitis, otitis, catarrh of eustachian tube, leucorrhoea, vulvo-vaginitis and balanitis.

ii. Energetic examination:

Lu. 1, l.	Left m. coracobrachialis
Sto. 25	Left hamstring muscles

23. **Penicillium piceum (penic-p.):**
   i. Pathology: Dyskinetic gallbladder.
   ii. Energetic examination:
CV 14	Hypertonic left m. subscapularis
Li. 14, bil.	Hypertonic left m. pectoralis major - pars sternalis
Li. 13, l.	Right m. latissimus dorsi
CV 3	Left m. peroneus longus and brevis

24. **Penicillium roqueforti (penic-r.):**
   i. Pathology: Loss of hair in men, offensive perspiring feet, frigidity in women.
   ii. Energetic examination:
CV 3	Left m. peroneus longus and brevis
Li. 13	Left m. trapezius, pars transversa
St. 25	Left m. quadratus lumborum

25. **Pityrosporum orbiculare (pityr-o.):**
   i. Pathology: Pityriasis versicolor
   ii. Energetic examination:
CV 4	Right m. quadratus femoris
CV 12	Left neck extensors
CV 17	Left m. gluteus medius
Li.13, r.	Left m. latissimus dorsi, not always present

26. **Rhizopus niger (rhiz.):**
   i. Pathology: Seborrhoea with alopecia in young age.
   ii. Energetic examination:
CV 3	Sacrospinalis m.: D 5 till D 12
CV 14	Right m. pectoralis minor

CV 17	Left m. soleus
Ha. 2, r.	Right m. teres major
St. 25, l. or r.	Left hamstring muscles

27. **Saccharomyces apiculata (sacmy-a.):**
  i. Pathology: Pityriasis versicolor
  ii. Energetic examination:

CV 3	Left or right m. tibialis anterior
Bl. 3, l.	Left m. supraspinatus, tested with little finger upward
Li. 13 (E.C.)	Left m. latissimus dorsi (E.C.)
St. 25, r.	

28. **Sporobolomyces roseus (sporob-r.):**
  i. Pathology: Nocturnal eneuresis, insufficiency of veins, varices.
  ii. Energetic examination:
  Sometimes there is a hemisphere switching: 1 / 1 ; 1 / 1 ; 1 / 1 ; ...

CV 3	Left and right m. peroneus tertius
CV 14	Left m. pectoralis minor
Li. 13, bil.	Right m. latissimus dorsi
N-LE 23	Left m. sartorius

  Triple Warmer 17, left.

29. **Sporobolomyces salmonicolor (sporob-s.):**
  i. Pathology: Acts on blood vessels causing arteriosclerosis, idiopathic hypertension and insufficiency of coronary arteries and heart.

ii. Energetic examination:

Li. 13, bil.	Right m. anconeus
	Left m. latissimus dorsi
St. 25, l.	Right m. quadratus lumborum

30. **Streptomyces citreus (actin-c.):** See, Actinomyces citreus
31. **Streptomyces griseus (actin-g.):** See, Actinomyces griseus
32. **Trichophyton depressum (trichoph-d.):**
    i. Pathology: Constipation*, seborrhoea with loss of hair, dandruff and itch.
    b. Energetic examination:

CV 3	Left m. peroneus longus and brevis
CV 12	Left m. sternocleidomastoideus
Ga. Bl. 25	Left or right m. psoas

    Weihe point of Phosphorus.

33. **Trichophyton persearum (trichoph-p.):**
    i. Pathology: Itching at soles of feet*, ringworm, intertrigo, eczema of swimmers.
    ii. Energetic examination:

Lu. 1, bil.	Left and/or right m. serratus anterior
C.-S. 2, r.	There is not a corresponding muscle till now

34. **Trichophyton rubrum (trichoph-r.):**
    i. Pathology: Ringworm, intertrigo (especially between toes), eczema of swimmers, psoriasis.
    ii. Energetic examination:

Sto. 25, l.	Left m. quadratus lumborum
Ga.Bl. 24	Left m. deltoideus anterior

Sub-type (code: 13737):

CV 12	Right m. pectoralis major - pars clavicularis*
Bl. 3, bil.	Right m. supraspinatus, tested with little finger upward*
Sto. 25, l.	Left m. quadratus lumborum *

35. **Trichophyton tonsurans (trichoph-t.):**
   i. Pathology: Seborrhoea with loss of hair.
   ii. Energetic examination:

CV 3	Left or right m. peroneus tertius
CV 5	Left m. teres minor and/or left m. infraspinatus
CV 12	Right m. sternocleidomastoideus right m. biceps
Li. 14	Right m. rhomboideus

RELATIONSHIP BETWEEN MUSCLE TESTS AND SOME HOMOEPATHIC REMEDIES OF BACTERIAL, VIRAL AND MYCOTIC ORIGIN

(Tested with eyes open in right-handed persons)

> **NB:**
> 1. If tested with eyes closed, the remedy is followed by (E.C.).
> 2. Homeopathic remedies from bacterial and viral origin are in normal print and homeopathic remedies from mycotic origin are printed in italics.
> 3. Remedies in bracket indicate that the lateralisation can be left or right, or alternate with another muscle.

1. Abdominals:
    i. Obliquus abdominis m. left internus / right externus (pushing into left direction): (aids), rota, (streptoc), (varic).
    ii. Obliquus abdominis m. right internus / left externus (pushing into right direction): (aids), molu., (streptoc), (varic).
2. Adductors
    i. Left: chlam., shigella-xyz.
    ii. Right: *asperg-fu.*, *asperg-n.*, brucel., (maland.)
3. Anconeus:
    i. Left: lyss., tetox.
       Hypertonic: diphtox.
    ii. Right: *sporob-s.*
4. Biceps brachii:
    i. Left: *anthraci.*, *fus.*, malar., *penic-cy.*, *trichoph-t.*

ii. Right: molu., parot.
5. Brachioradialis:
   i. Left: borre-b.
   ii. Right: *asperg-br.*
6. Cloacals:
   i. Anterior ipsilateral cloacal: pyrog.
   ii. Anterior contralateral cloacal: chlam.
7. Coracobrachialis:
   i. Left: *fus.*, maland., meningoc-vc., *penic-n.*
   ii. Right:
8. Deltoideus anterior:
   i. Left : (brucel.), chlam., hippoz., oscilloc., *penic-can.*, rota, *trichoph-r.*, urpl-ul.
   ii. Right: (brucel.), *moni.*, toxo-g.
9. Deltoideus medius:
   i. Left: aids, (hippoz.), influ., prot-mir., pyrog.
      Hypertonic: ccv-xyz.
   ii. Right: eberth., eps-b.
10. Deltoideus posterior:
    i. Left: (hippoz.), maland., staphycoc.
    ii. Right:
11. Fascia lata:
    i. Left: (chlam.), coli., (cytom-v.), lyss., polio-vc-sn., rota, (streptoc.), (varic.)
       Hypertonic: parapert.
    ii. Right: (chlam.), (cytom-v.), (streptoc.), (varic.)
12. Gluteus maximus:
    i. Left: *asperg-n.*, borre-b., *fus.*, helico-p., maland., (*moni.*), (pert.), (polio-vc-sn.)

ii. Right: bact-fr., coli., eberth., (*moni.*), *mucor*, mucot-kp., (pert.), (polio-vc-sn.), scarl., vac.
13. Gluteus medius:
    i. Left: (aids), *asperg-fu.*, (brucel.), ccv-xyz., cytom-v., (influ.), mucot-kp., (streptoc.), (tetox.)
    ii. Right: (aids), *asperg-n.*, (brucel.), hippoz., (influ.), *penic-chr.*, (streptoc.), (tetox.), varic.
14. Gracilis:
    i. Left: mycopl-pn., (pyrog.), tetox.
    ii. Right: aids, (maland.), (pyrog.), toxo-g.
15. Hamstrings:
    i. Left: (brucel.), (cytom-v.), maland., *penic-n., rhiz.,* yell-vc.
    ii. Right: (brucel.), (cytom-v.), hippoz., scarl.
16. Iliacus:
    i. Left: (*asperg-br.*), malar.
    ii. Right: (*asperg-br.*)
17. Infraspinatus:
    i. Left: chlam., (rs-v.), (toxo-g.), *trichoph-t.*
    ii. Right: clostri-pf., eberth., (rs-v.), (toxo-g.)
18. Latissimus dorsi:
    i. Left: *actin-c., actin-l.*, chlam., *clados-m.*, (*moni.*), (mucot-kp.), helico-p., influ., mycopl-pn., *penic-can., sacmy-a.* (*E.C.*), *sporob-s.*, (staphycoc.), staphyloc-a (vario.).
    Hypertonic: prevo-im.
    ii. Right: aids, (*moni.*), (mucot-kp.), *penic-p., sporob-r.*, (staphycoc.) (vario.).
19. Levator scapulae:
    i. Left:
    ii. Right: polio-vc-sn.
20. Neck extensors:
    i. Left: parot.

ii. Right: parot.
21. Neck flexors:
   Sternocleidomastoideus m.:
   i. Left: *actin-c.*, (chlam.), *clados-m.*, helico-p., mucoc., staphycoc., (strepto.), *trichoph-d.*, yell-vc.
      Hypertonic: mucot-mt.
   ii. Right: (chlam.), *penic-chr.*, *trichoph-t.*
22. Pectoralis major - pars clavicularis:
   i. Left: anthraci., barto-h., diphtox.
      Hypertonic: enteroc., influ-co., myco-gn.
   ii. Right: aids, scarl., streptoc., *trichoph-r.**
      Hypertonic: influ-co.
23. Pectoralis major - pars sternalis:
   i. Left: (hippoz.), (influ.), malar., staphyloc-a., (vac.), varic.
      Hypertonic: enteroc., *penic-p.*
   ii. Right: bact-fr., barto-h., eberth., herp-s., (hippoz.), (influ.), mucot-mt., parapert., polio-vc-sn., (vac.)
      Hypertonic: shigella-xyz.
24. Pectoralis minor:
   i. Left: (chlam.), (dysentery), eberth., *sporob-r.*
   ii. Right: (chlam.), (dysentery), *rhiz.*, staphycoc., vac.
      Hypertonic: prevo-im.
25. Peroneus longus and brevis:
   i. Left: (aids), chlam., *clados-m., fus.,* parot., *penic-p., penic-r., trichoph-d.*
   ii. Right: *aclad.*, (aids), *(asperg-br.), penic-cy.*, prevo-im., polio-vc-sn.
26. Peroneus tertius:
   i. Left: herp-g., hippoz., *(moni.)*, mucoc., *mucor*, (rs-v.), *sporob-r.*

       Hypertonic: (rs-v.)
    ii. Right: (*moni.*), *sporob-r.*
27. Piriformis:
    i. Left: cytom-v., (pert.)
    ii. Right: (pert.)
28. Popliteus:
    i. Left: aids, morb., general anesthetics (especially fentanyl), mucoc.
    ii. Right: *clados-m.*, dysentery, polio-vc-sn.
29. Pronator teres
    i. Left: enteroc.
    ii. Right:
30. Psoas:
    i. Left: (*asperg-br.*), coli., (*trichoph-d.*), (varic.)
       Hypertonic:
    ii. Right: (*asperg-br.*), maland., (*trichoph-d.*), (varic.)
       Hypertonic: (oscilloc. – E.C.)
31. Pterygoideus internus (medialis):
    i. Left: enteroc.
    ii. Right:
32. Quadratus lumborum:
    i. Left: *actin-c.*, bact-fr., borre-b., (chlam.), cytom-v., *mucor*, *penic-r.*, (prot-mir.), rota, (tetox.), *trichoph-r., trichoph-r.**, yell-vc.
       Hypertonic:
    ii. Right: (chlam.), polio-vc-sn., (prot-mir.), *sporob-s.*, staphycoc., (tetox.)
       Hypertonic: streptoc.

33. Quadriceps femoris:
    i. Left: *actin-c., actin-g.*, borre-b., (dysentery), maland., *penic-e. (E.C)*, (toxo-g.)
        Hypertonic:
    ii. Right: (dysentery), helico-p., herp-s., *penic-chr.*, polio-vc-sn., (toxo-g.)
        Hypertonic: myco-gn.
34. Rhomboideus:
    i. Left: (mucot-kp.), hepati-b-vc., molu., oscilloc., *penic-chr.*, (prot-mir.), pyrog., (varic.)
        Hypertonic: ccv-xyz., clostri-pf., (hepati-a-vc.)
    ii. Right: *aclad.*, bact-fr., coli., (mucot-kp.), *penic-can., penic-cy.*, (prot-mir.), *trichoph-t.*, (varic.)
        Hypertonic: (hepati-a-vc.)
35. Sacrospinalis: (*asperg-br.*), meningoc-vc.
    i. D1 – D12 : toxo-g.
    ii. D5 – D12: *rhiz.*
36. Sartorius:
    i. Left: (varic.), (*trichoph-p.*)
    ii. Right: (*trichoph-p.*), (varic.)
37. Serratus anterior:
    i. Left: maland., morb., (pert.), *thrichoph-p.*, vario.
    ii. Right: *asperg-fu.*, mucot-kp., *thrichoph-p.*
38. Soleus:
    i. Left: *rhiz.*
    ii. Right:
39. Subscapularis, hand near chest:
    i. Left: *actin-g.*, (aids), (influ.), (*moni.*), mucor, (mucot-kp.), polio-vc-sn., vario.

Hypertonic: *penic-p.*
  ii. Right: (aids), (influ.), (*moni.*), (mucot-kp.), urpl-ul.
40. Supraspinatus, hand facing toward the body:
  i. Left: (brucel.), (oscilloc. – E.C.), (streptoc.), vac., (varic.)
  ii. Right: aids, (brucel.), eberth., lyss., oscilloc., polio-vc-sn., (streptoc.), (varic.)
41. Supraspinatus, little finger upward (pronation):
  i. Left: (chlam.), diphtox., herp-s., influ., *sacmy-a.*
  ii. Right: aids, borre-b., (chlam.), eps-b., helico-p., *penic-e.*, rs-v., tetox., *trichoph-r.**, urpl-ul.
  iii. Left and right, simultaneously: varic.
42. Supraspinatus, thumb upward (supination):
  i. Left: anthraci., *actin-l.*, dysentery, herp-g.
  ii. Right: *aleur-l. (E.C)*, hepati-a-vc., hepati-b-vc., mucot-mc.
43. Teres major:
  i. Left: *penic-g.*, (staphycoc.), (urpl-ul)., vario., yell-vc.
  Hypertonic: (urpl-ul.)
  ii. Right: brucel., mucoc., *rhiz.*, (staphycoc.)
  Hypertonic: influ-A/H_1N_1
44. Teres minor:
  i. Left: brucel., (staphyloc-a.), (toxo-g.), *trichoph-t.*, varic.
  ii. Right: aids, hippoz., maland., staphycoc., (staphyloc-a.), (toxo-g.)
45. Tibialis anterior:
  i. Left: (brucel.), *(sacmy-a.)*
  ii. Right: (brucel.), *(sacmy-a.)*, tetox.
46. Trapezius, upper:
  i. Left: lyss.

Hypertonic: hepati-b-vc.
ii. Right:
Hypertonic: hepati-a-vc.
47. Trapezius, middle:
   i. Left: (dysentery), meningoc-vc., *penic-r.*
      Hypertonic:
   ii. Right: (dysentery)
48. Trapezius, lower:
   i. Left: (aids), (brucel.), *penic-g.*, (pert.)
   ii. Right: (aids), (brucel.), eps-b., (pert.)
49. Triceps brachii:
   i. Left: barto-h., ccv-xyz., *penic-chr.*
   ii. Right:

CONCLUSION

Miasms are dynamic forces 'in evolution' which are in connection with all energies all over the world and even the universe. They consist of different layers, each having a special correspondence to some energy.

The pure energy is in the centre and is connected with the energy of the universe. The psychological energy is especially connected with the archetypes, the emotional energy with water and stars and the physical energy with the earth and sun.

The quick multiplication and evolution of bacteria, viruses and yeasts form the dynamic power of the evolution of all other species on earth because it obliges them to adapt and evolve. This evolution also touches the centre of each miasm.

That's why the homeopathic application of nosodes is so important. They make very essential energetic corrections which have positive repercussions on the immune system.

Appendix

Handmode Figures

Figures with the specific finger positions concerning the handmodes:

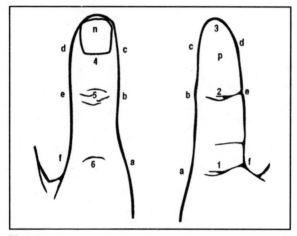

Thumb

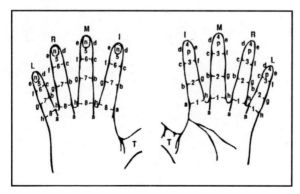

Hands

Bibliography

ACUPUNCTURE

Essentials of Chinese Acupuncture, compiled by Beijing, Shanghai, Nanjing College of traditional Chinese Medicine and the Acupuncture Institute of the Academy of Traditional Chinese Medicine, Beijing: Foreign Languages Press, 1980.

HOMEOPATHY

1. Agrawal, Y.R., A Treatise on Bowel Nosodes, Delhi: Vijay Publications, 1981.
2. Allen, J.H., The Chronic Miasms, Vol. I: Psora and Pseudopsora and Vol. II: Sycosis, Delhi: B. Jain Publishers, 1981.
3. Allen, H.C., The Materia Medica of the Nosodes, Delhi: B. Jain Publishers.
4. Allen, T.F., The Encyclopedia of Pure Materia Medica (12 vol.), Vaduz: The Gregg Press Establish.
5. Barthel, H. & Klunker, W., Synthetic Repertory (3 vol.), Heidelberg: Karl Haug Verlag, 2nd ed., 1982.
6. Bernard, H., Traité de médecine homéopathique, Harz: Laboratoire Unda, 3rd éd., 1985.
7. Bjorndal, A., Towards an Unified Homeopathy, The system of miasms, 2003, Norsk Akademi for Naturmedisin.

8. Boericke, W. & O., Homoeopathic Materia Medica with Repertory, London: Homoeopathic Book Service, 1st Brit. ed., 1987.
9. Boger, C.M., Boenninghausen's Characteristics and Repertory, Delhi: B. Jain Publishers, 1984.
10. Cicchetti, J., Dreams, Symbols, & Homoeopathy, North Atlantic Books, Berkeley, California, 2003.
11. Chand, D.H., Cancerinic or cancerinic state, Delhi: National Homoeopathic Pharmacy, 1981.
12. Clarke, J. H., A Dictionary of Practical Materia Medica, (3 vol.), Bradford: Health Science Press, 3rd ed., 1977.
13. Degroote, F., Carcinosinum, Eeklo: H.R.I.C., 1986.
14. Degroote, F., Physical Examination and Observations in Homoeopathy, Gent: Homeoden/Heel Book service, 1992.
15. Degroote, F., Dromen vanuit homeopathisch perspectief, Bruges, 2004.
16. Farrington, E.A., Comparative Materia Medica, Delhi: B. Jain Publishers, 1980.
17. Hahnemann, S., Materia Medica Pura (2 vol.), Delhi: B. Jain Publishers, 1983.
18. Hahnemann, S., Les maladies chroniques (translated by P. Schmidt and J. Künzli), Paris: Maisonneuve, 3rd éd. fr., 1969.
19. Hering, C., The guiding symptoms of our Materia Medica, (10 vol.), Delhi: B. Jain Publishers, 1983.
20. Julian, O.A., Dictionnaire de matière médicale homéopathique, Paris: Editions Masson, 1981.
21. Kent, J.T., Lectures on Homoeopathic Materia Medica, Philadelphia: Boericke & Tafel, 4th ed., 1946.
22. Kent, J.T., New remedies, Clinical cases, Lesser writings, Aphorisms and Precepts, Delhi: B. Jain Publishers, 1981.

23. Kent, J.T., Repertory of the Homoeopathic Materia Medica, Sittingbourne: Homoeopathic Book Service, 2nd Brit. ed., 1990.
24. Masi, A., Cours supérieur de révision de la doctrine de la technique de de la matière médicale homéopathique, Gent: Homeoden Book Service, 1989.
25. Ortega, P.S., Notes on the Miasms.
26. Paterson, J., The Bowel Nosodes, The British Homoeopathic Journal, Vol. XL (1950), Nth 3.
27. Roberts, H.A., The Principles and Art of Cure by Homoeopathy, Delhi: B. Jain Publishers, 1981.
28. Sankaran, R., The Spirit of Homoeopathy, Bombay: Homoeopathic Medical Publishers, 1992.
29. Sankaran, R., The Substance of Homoeopathy, Bombay: Homoeopathic Medical Publishers, 1994.
30. Van der Zee, H., Miasms in labour, Utrecht : Stichting Alonnissos, 2000.
31. Vannier, L., Les cancériniques et leur traitement homéopathiques, Paris : G.Doin & Cie Editeurs, Paris, 1952.
32. Vannier, L. and Poirier, J., Précis de matière homéopathique, Paris: Doin éditions, 9th éd., 1981.

KINESIOLOGY

1. Beardall, A.G., Clinical Kinesiology, Portland: Human Bio-Dynamics, 1990.
2. Walther, D.S., Applied Kinesiology, Synopsis, Colorado: Systems DC, 1988.

Index of Cases

1. Agaricus muscarius : 81, 82
2. Allium cepa : 29, 30
3. Astacus fluviatilis : 82, 83, 84
4. Calcarea carbonicum : 20, 31, 47, 77, 92, 105, 113
5. Calcarea phosphorica : 20, 47, 92
6. Carcinosinum : 20, 21, 48, 57, 71, 73, 74, 76, 77, 78, 79, 81, 86, 88, 89, 91, 94, 95, 96, 97, 99, 108, 120, 121, 122, 147, 148, 149, 162, 163, 166
7. Cisplatina : 84, 123, 124
8. Kalium phosphoricum : 47, 74, 75, 76
9. Lac caninum : 80, 81
10. Lycopodium clavatum : 20, 23, 34, 35, 78, 79, 91, 122, 137, 141
11. Medorrhinum : 20, 27, 33, 34, 47, 54, 57, 71, 77, 78, 79, 82, 83, 84, 85, 86, 89, 90, 92, 94, 95, 98, 99, 100, 108, 115, 116, 117, 118, 119, 133, 162, 163, 166, 171, 174
12. Morgan-Gartnaer (Paterson) : 24, 25, 35, 126, 127, 130, 136, 137, 154, 155, 156, 157, 158, 159, 161
13. Nux vomica : 19, 20, 31, 32, 42, 58, 59, 80, 130, 131, 132

14. Psorinum : 20, 27, 39, 47, 57, 73, 74, 75, 85, 86, 87, 88, 95, 99, 108, 109, 110, 112, 113, 114, 157, 158, 159, 160, 161, 166, 167, 171

15. Staphysagria : 33, 34

16. Sulphur : 20, 29, 30, 113, 130

17. Syphilinum : 20, 27, 31, 33, 47, 57, 71, 85, 89, 91, 93, 94, 95, 99, 100, 102, 108, 119, 120, 146, 150, 162, 163, 166

18. Tuberculinum : 20, 27, 31, 47, 57, 71, 77, 78, 79, 81, 82, 84, 85, 90, 91, 93, 94, 95, 101, 102, 103, 104, 105, 106, 108, 123, 124, 144, 162, 164, 166, 173, 182

19. Zincum metallicum : 77